Praise for Sex and the Single Girl

Sex and the Single Girl is the best resource I know of how to embrace the idea that women are sexual, but not stay stuck in delayed longings or desires we don't know what to do with. Juli Slattery has created a resource that will help you walk through your sexuality as God intends, without leaving you feeling like you are left alone to figure things out on your own. As we are living in a sexually confused culture, let Juli be your mentor and guide.

ESTHER FLEECE
Speaker, author of *No More Faking Fine*

In a world where sex is ubiquitous, I don't think we're even really talking about it. Not real sex, anyway. This book will fuel the conversation. Every college Bible study group and every singles group should be using this fantastic book to enlighten women about the purpose and practices of sex. Juli creates an amazing, conversational atmosphere with this study that will fuel transparent and soul-healing conversations among single women. She's unafraid to speak black-and-white truth. Equally as important, she admits that there are some gray areas when it comes to truth about sex. Dive in and be a part of the conversation.

DANNAH GRESH
Author *And the Bride Wore White* and *What Are You Waiting For?*

In a generation of young women who are struggling to understand God's design for sexuality, this book is a must-read. Seriously—every young woman needs to get her hands on a copy of *Sex and the Single Girl*. This powerful resource is biblical, practical, down-to-earth, and incredibly easy to read. It will transform your perspective on sexuality and get you excited about God's beautiful design.

KRISTEN CLARK AND BETHANY BAIRD
Founders of GirlDefined Ministries
Authors of *Girl Defined: God's Radical Design for Beauty, Femininity, and Identity*

Young women today are bombarded by a sexual message that will not give them the intimacy they long for. If they step onto a college campus prepped only with a "sex is wrong" mindset, they won't make it. In order to face the immense pressure, they must be convinced that there is something better out there than what the culture offers. Thank you, Juli, for providing single women with the knowledge and understanding to help them hold out for God's best. This is a must-read for every college student.

KIM VOLLENDORF
Regional leader, StuMo Campus ministry
Author of *Loving Your Husband Before You Even Have One* (January 2018)

Juli's study is not a list of dos and don'ts, but an invitation to consider what the Bible says about sexuality and draw near to the loving God who created us to be sexual beings. Regardless of your past, you are welcome here! As a woman who disciples younger women, I appreciate the clarity and hope with which Juli encourages a life of sexual integrity. *Sex and the Single Girl* is a helpful and encouraging guide for exploring truth about sexuality.

LISA SANDQUIST
Codirector of The Navigators Global Student Program

Sex and the Single Girl is an invaluable resource for women whether single, dating, or engaged (and even married)! Christian women on college campuses are desperate for a resource like this to serve as a framework for understanding and engaging with our sexuality. We cannot ignore that we are sexual beings. *Sex and the Single Girl* gives permission for us to know ourselves as such. As a Christian woman in ministry, I am often unsatisfied with how we engage this topic and I am looking for ways to support and guide my students as they navigate their sexuality. This book offers these opportunities. I'm incredibly thankful.

SARAH YOUSSEF
Residence Supervisor

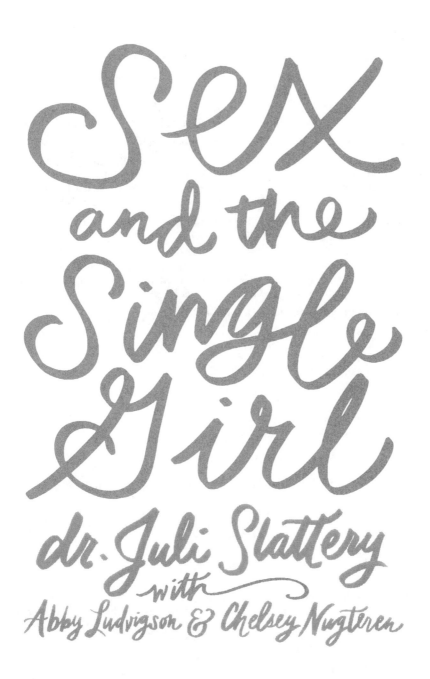

Sex and the Single Girl

dr. Juli Slattery

with

Abby Ludvigson & Chelsey Nugteren

MOODY PUBLISHERS

CHICAGO

All Scripture quotations, unless otherwise indicated, are taken from the Holy Bible, New International Version®, NIV®. Copyright © 1973, 1978, 1984, 2011 by Biblica, Inc.™ Used by permission of Zondervan. All rights reserved worldwide. www.zondervan.com. The "NIV" and "New International Version" are trademarks registered in the United States Patent and Trademark Office by Biblica, Inc.™

Scripture quotations marked ESV are from The Holy Bible, English Standard Version® (ESV®), copyright © 2001 by Crossway, a publishing ministry of Good News Publishers. Used by permission. All rights reserved.

Scripture quotations marked NLT are taken from the Holy Bible, New Living Translation, copyright © 1996, 2004, 2007, 2013 by Tyndale House Foundation. Used by permission of Tyndale House Publishers, Inc., Carol Stream, Illinois 60188. All rights reserved.

Emphasis in Scripture quotations has been added by the author.

Edited by Linda Joy Neufeld
Cover design: Connie Gabbert Design and Illustration
Interior design: Smartt Guys design
Author photo: Kandid Kate Photography

Library of Congress Cataloging-in-Publication Data

Names: Slattery, Julianna, 1969- author.
Title: Sex and the single girl / Dr. Juli Slattery, with Abby Ludvigson &
  Chelsey Nugteren.
Description: Chicago : Moody Publishers, 2017. | Includes bibliographical
  references.
Identifiers: LCCN 2017019914 (print) | LCCN 2017027168 (ebook) | ISBN
  9780802496324 ISBN 9780802416742
Subjects: LCSH: Christian women--Religious life. | Sex--Religious
  aspects--Christianity. | Single people--Sexual behavior.
Classification: LCC BV4527 (ebook) | LCC BV4527 .S495 2017 (print) | DDC
  241/.664082--dc23
LC record available at https://lccn.loc.gov/2017019914

We hope you enjoy this book from Moody Publishers. Our goal is to provide high-quality, thought-provoking books and products that connect truth to your real needs and challenges. For more information on other books and products written and produced from a biblical perspective, go to www.moodypublishers.com or write to:

Moody Publishers
820 N. LaSalle Boulevard
Chicago, IL 60610

1 3 5 7 9 10 8 6 4 2

Printed in the United States of America

Chelsey, thank you for all of the groups you took through different versions of this study. Your input and feedback have been invaluable. Abby, you took my "wad of gum" and stretched it out into a teachable format that women can grasp! This was a team effort and I'm thankful for your contributions.

Contents

Note from Juli 8

Week 1: Why Sexuality Matters 12

Week 2: Embracing a Grand Design 34

Week 3: Sexuality and Your Character 58

Week 4: Sexual Boundaries 82

Week 5: Battling Temptation 100

Week 6: Restoring Intimacy with God 124

Now What? 144

Notes 147

Acknowledgments 148

About the Author 149

Note from Juli

Welcome to *Sex and the Single Girl*! I'm thrilled that you've decided to dive into this study (or even just put your big toe in the water to check it out). A lot of time, work, and prayer has gone into this study. Why? Because I know that sexuality is a very loaded and emotional topic. I know how confusing and shame inducing it can be to talk about things like sex, cohabitation, porn, masturbation, and LGBT issues. But I also know that women like you are seeking truth and hope for your own journey through the minefield of sexuality.

I don't promise to have the answers to every question you might ask, but I'm committed to seeking truth alongside you. Through this study, you can expect to be challenged, to learn some things you've never heard before and to perhaps realize for the first time that God cares about every aspect of your life, including your sexuality.

You won't get far into the study before you begin to see that I view sexuality as a spiritual battlefield. God has an enemy and so do you. Satan has an agenda to twist and distort everything that God has created as holy. As we look around the landscape of our world, sexuality appears to be in Satan's bull's-eye. While God created your sexuality to be a blessing, most women experience it as tainted and filled with shame.

The perspective throughout this study is going to be quite different from what you might be hearing from friends and even your college professors. Everyone has an opinion on sexual issues. My hope and prayer is that you don't get *my opinion*, but that you learn to seek God's opinion. And you know what we call God's opinion: truth. He is the Creator of sexuality, and He alone knows the purpose for which He designed it.

Because sexuality is a spiritual battlefield, you need to approach this study keeping that in mind. There are many voices in the world. The only one that truly matters is God's voice. God promises, "I will instruct and teach you in the way you should go" (Ps. 32:8), but we must learn to listen.

The best way to listen to God is to regularly set aside time to study, to pray, to journal, and just to hear God's voice to you. Far too many women settle for secondhand information about a very personal God. I don't want to just tell you about God, I want to encourage you to personally seek Him and know Him. God said, "You will seek me and find me when you seek me with all your heart" (Jer. 29:13). The best way to seek the Lord is to find a time, find a place, and find a plan. During this season of my life, my time with God usually looks like this:

Time: 5:00 a.m.
Place: In my living room by my fireplace
Plan: I spend time in worship/prayer and then read the 1-year Bible plan

I might have just turned you off by sharing my time, place, and plan. When I was in college, a 5:00 a.m. time with God would have resulted in me drooling on my Bible. And reading through the Bible in a year would have intimidated me. I'm at a different stage of life as a mom of three teenage boys. You pick your time, your place, and your plan. Make it work for the season of life you're in now! Maybe your best time of day is 10:00 p.m. in your bedroom. Maybe this study will be your "plan" for the next several weeks. Whatever works best for you. The point is to take time to spend with God.

GETTING THE MOST FROM THIS STUDY

As I mentioned earlier, the perspective of sexuality you're about to read may be very different from what you're hearing from friends, professors, and the culture around you. That means this information will likely be new to you. The best way to digest new thoughts and ideas is to stop and react to what you've read by marking up the book. Over the course of the next six weeks, I want to challenge you to interact with this study rather than mindlessly read the words. Engage with it, ask questions, be surprised, be honest. Below are common markings you can use to remember a thought so you can follow up on it later. You can complete this study by yourself or with a group. The study is broken into six weeks with five days of homework per week. It will probably take you about 15 minutes to complete each day's study. Some groups found it helpful to stretch the study out for 12 weeks to allow for more discussion and less pressure to get the homework done. Feel free to adapt the structure of the book to your own schedule and to your group's needs.

! = this surprised me

? = I don't understand

L = I learned something new

♡ = this touched my heart

As you read, you will see a few stopping points to remind you to absorb and apply what you are learning. You will see both "Reflect and Respond" and "Now It's Your Turn" questions. These questions are designed to encourage you to stop and digest what you just read and personalize it to your own life. God has a lot He wants to teach you but if you're not willing to engage with Him you will become lost in how to apply what you are learning. You will also notice comments and testimonies from women throughout the study. These are real testimonies of women just like you as they went through the pilot study. Many of their names have been changed, but their thoughts have been recorded just as they wrote them.

HELPFUL ADDITIONS

You will notice each week we've added questions at the beginning and then summary statements at the end. The purpose is to highlight the concepts we want you to take away with you. The "Have You Ever Asked Yourself" Questions will give you a heads-up on the kind of questions we will address each week. The summary statements at the end will take everything you've learned that week and put it into takeaway sentences that are easier to remember.

DIGGING DEEPER RESOURCES

As you are going through this study, you might find a topic that hits a nerve for you. Maybe you want to dig deeper into an issue you are currently struggling with, like recovering from abuse or kicking a porn habit. The *Sex and the Single Girl* study is just one resource from the ministry Authentic Intimacy. At www.authenticintimacy.com, you will find blogs, podcasts, and much more to help you learn more about specific areas of sexuality. I'd also encourage you to go through this study with a group of other women. You will be encouraged to know that they can relate to your questions and struggles.

ONE LAST THING

I realize that you may be coming to this study with difficult things in your past. Sexuality is a topic that makes us curious, but can also surface feelings of fear, shame, and sadness. Maybe you are one of the 20 percent of women who have experienced sexual abuse in childhood. If you are, my heart grieves with you and I pray that this study will be part of your healing journey. Perhaps you have made sexual choices that you regret. You wonder how God views you in light of your choices or your current temptations. Although we have probably never met, I know that God has you on His heart. So thank you for your bravery in picking up *Sex and the Single Girl*.

I want you to know that we ALL have experienced sexual brokenness of some sort. You are among friends who can understand your journey and identify with your fears. Most importantly, Jesus knows exactly how you feel. As you stand at the door of this study, please know that He is not a condemning Judge but a welcoming Savior. He died to set each one of us, including *you*, free from sin, shame, and condemnation.

If you read something in this study that brings up pain or shame, please tell a trusted friend (maybe someone in the group). But most importantly, please tell the Lord. God is a God of comfort, compassion, and presence. My prayer for you during this study is that you come to know Him in a more powerful and personal way.

Okay, friend. Are you ready? Let's dive in . . .

Why

Have you ever asked yourself . . .

- *Why do many women separate their sexuality from their faith?*
- *What does it mean to be a sexual woman?*
- *Is there a deeper purpose underneath my sexuality than just having sex?*
- *What does my sexuality reveal about me and why did God design me that way?*
- *How does my sexuality paint a picture of the gospel?*
- *On what truth do most people base their sexual choices?*
- *Are my sexuality and my spiritual identity separate or do they align?*

This week's study, "Why Sexuality Matters," will bring you clarity on these questions and more.

Sexuality Matters

Who Taught You about Sex?

"I was raised to believe that sex is something you wait for until marriage. But God hasn't brought marriage, and no one around me seems to think that God cares about me waiting. Does God really want me to have all these desires and nowhere to go with them? Really? How long does He expect me to wait?"

"I'm a Christian but I don't agree with a lot of what the Bible says about sex. Sex is about love, isn't it? So why would God care if two women love each other sexually?"

"Whenever I hear people talk about purity, I tune out. I've already been with guys so none of this even relates to me anymore."

"I have yet to meet a guy who doesn't want to have sex within the first few months of dating. It's just assumed that dating means sex, even with guys who say they are Christians. It's a different world than when my parents grew up."

I'm guessing that you can relate to what these women are wrestling with. We live in a sexually chaotic world. There are no standards other than *be true to yourself* and *don't judge anyone else's sexual choices.* And sex is *everywhere.* There is hardly a sitcom or movie that doesn't have strong sexual themes. The daily headlines are filled with reports of sexual scandals, the impact of changing laws, and personal sexual freedom.

And then there's you . . . your life. You have your own private battles. We've heard from many women like you who share some of the pressures and challenges you face.

Maybe you carry with you sexual secrets you would never share with anyone and the shame from your past haunts you. Or maybe you don't know what the big deal is about sex. Does God really care if you sleep around, look at porn, or experiment with another woman sexually? Doesn't He want you to be happy?

There is probably no topic that creates more confusion or pain than sexuality. The questions above are just the tip of the iceberg. Many women have sexual abuse in their past; others equate their sexuality with guilt and shame. And most Christian sources haven't been very helpful in sorting through the deep questions women are asking.

REFLECT AND RESPOND

- *What pressures and challenges are you, your roommate, and/or close friends battling right now?*

- *What questions are you having a hard time sorting through on your own?*

- *How would you like your life to be different after going through this study?*

YOU GOT YOUR OPINIONS FROM SOMEWHERE

Think for a moment about what you learned about sexuality from your parents. How about from church or Christian books? Was there silence or could you honestly ask questions about masturbation, boundaries in dating, and what being a "virgin" really means? We are typically pretty clumsy and reserved in teaching a Christian view of sex. If you grew up in church, maybe all you ever heard was "Don't do it . . . until you get married."

While most parents and church leaders seem to be uncomfortable talking about sexuality, the culture has no problem inserting the topic into almost every venue. Because of this disparity, even a woman who loves God may have a difficult time understanding how her sexuality relates to her faith. Sex just seems too personal and crude for God to care much about. While we may orient other parts of life to what God wants, our sexuality seems like a separate category.

God wants all of your life to be in agreement with His design for you. Why? Because He knows what is best for you. Unfortunately, the average woman has been given very little (maybe no) teaching on sexuality from a biblical perspective. Even the most committed

Christian often thinks about sexual issues from a worldly mindset. Through *Sex and the Single Girl* we want to change that. I'd like to show you how your love for God and His love for you can deeply impact the choices you make and the beliefs you hold about sexuality.

> My mom didn't talk to us much that I remember but I do recall her telling us that if we ever decided to have sex, it was no big deal. She would buy whatever we needed to be protected—as in birth control, condoms, etc. My dad on the other hand gave me a very messed up idea. He had, or rather has, an extensive *Playboy* collection. He doesn't see anything wrong in it and in fact would argue the value of them. I don't think my mom wanted us to know about the magazines, but since he kept a few in the house we found them. His porn use made me believe that sex is dirty and that a woman's value is only in her sexuality, how she portrays herself, and giving herself to a man. —Jenna

> Sex was never mentioned in our house, besides that one awkward conversation I had with my mom when I turned thirteen. I had no one to ask questions to and no safe place to discuss things I was experiencing. Because of this I turned to friends and the Internet. I felt so much shame for even feeling attracted to boys because the only message I ever heard was "Sex is bad." —Mallory

REFLECT AND RESPOND

- *What percentage of your thinking about sex came from your parents? Religious teaching? Media? Other sources?*

Parents _____%   Religion _____%   Media _____%   Other _____%

- *What are the primary things you've learned about sex from each of these sources?*

Parents:

Religion:

Media:

Other:

• Do you agree that it's difficult to understand how your sexuality relates to your faith? Why or why not?

• Think about the last twenty-four hours. What messages has the culture shared about sexuality? (Think of the shows you watch, music you listen to, etc.) Write down some of the messages you've heard in the past twenty-four hours from these three sources:

TV:

Music:

Social media:

Sex Is a Brilliant Metaphor of a Profound Truth

Let's begin with the truth that you are a sexual woman. Even if you have never had sex or are currently not sexually active, you are still a sexual person. To take that a step further, you are sexual *by God's design*. He intentionally created you female, with the physical anatomy and biochemical properties of sexuality. This means that you have longings for intimacy, relationship, *and* physical pleasure.

You don't magically become a sexual person when you have sex or when you get married. The expression of your sexuality changes under these circumstances, but you have always been a sexual person.

Sex, sexuality, and intimacy are often used interchangeably in our culture. This makes the whole discussion even more confusing. Your sexuality involves more than just having sex. Your desire for intimacy transcends your desire for sex. Throughout this study, keep the following definitions in mind:

Sexuality: A broad concept encompassing all aspects of a person's gender, sexual desire, sexual beliefs, and sexual experiences.

Intimacy: A close, familiar, and usually affectionate or loving personal relationship with another person. Intimacy involves the experience of safety, vulnerability, and being deeply known.

Sex: Physical activity that is related to and often includes sexual intercourse.

Why the distinction? Because our culture talks endlessly about the act of sex but ignores the bigger picture of sexuality. Christian teachers may give guidelines about "how far is too far," but typically avoid the deeper questions related to what it means to be single and sexual. As a single woman, you may not be having sex, but your sexuality deeply impacts many aspects of your life.

To understand the importance of your sexuality, you have to grasp that sex is first and foremost a brilliant metaphor of a profound truth (a *metaphor* is a figure of speech which compares two things that are unrelated but share some common characteristics). Underneath your sexuality is the drive and desire to be known and loved. God created you as a sexual being so that you might understand what it means to long, to desire, and to crave intimate oneness. Your sexuality was never meant to be an isolated physiological urge that is expressed apart from the rest of who you are as a woman. You have longings to share your heart, soul, and body with another person because God made you a deeply relational and spiritual woman. Your greatest need for intimacy however is to know the God who created you.

Does that seem farfetched? Here is one example of why we can say this with confidence. The first part of the Bible (called the Old Testament) was written in Hebrew. The Hebrew word for sexual intimacy between a husband and wife used in the Old Testament is *yada*. The first time this word, *yada*, is used in the Bible is right here:

> Now Adam knew [*yada*] his wife Eve, and she conceived and bore Cain . . . . Cain knew [*yada*] his wife, and she conceived and bore Enoch. . . . And Adam knew [*yada*] his wife again, and she bore a son and called his name Seth. (Gen. 4:1, 17, 25 ESV, emphasis mine)

Yada literally means "to know deeply or intimately." This Hebrew word, *yada*, is in the Old Testament over 940 times. Most of the time, the word *yada* is not referring to sex but used to describe intimacy with God—His with us and ours with Him. Here are a few examples:

> You have searched me, Lord, and you [*yada*] me. (Ps. 139:1, emphasis mine)

In all your ways [*yada*] to Him, and He will make your paths straight. (Prov. 3:6, emphasis mine)

Moses said to the Lord, "If you are pleased with me, teach me your ways so I may [*yada*] you and continue to find favor with you." (Ex. 33:12–13, emphasis mine)

Take a minute now and go back to each of these verses. Underneath the verse, rewrite the verse but this time with the definition of *yada* in place of the actual word *yada*. (Example: You have searched me and you [intimately know] my heart.)

Why would God inspire the authors of the Bible to use a word related to sexual intimacy to also describe His relationship with His people? Because marriage and sexuality were always intended to teach us about intimacy with God.

Sexuality is a powerful picture of God's invitation to intimacy. The physical longings related to your sexuality point to a much deeper, more profound longing to be known intimately. We live in a culture that consistently tries to separate sex from all it was intended to express. While sexuality was designed to be a wonderful expression of intimacy, it has become a cheap replacement for it. We live in a culture that discourages long-term relationships, trust, and emotional intimacy. The prevailing message is that physical nakedness can fulfill your desire for true intimacy. The prevailing message is wrong.

REFLECT AND RESPOND

- *When you think of the word intimacy, what first comes to mind? How does this brief teaching expand your understanding of intimacy?*

- *Is the concept that underneath your sexuality there is a drive and desire to be known and loved revolutionary to you? If so, why? If not, why not?*

• *Read Psalm 139, a psalm of intimate knowing. The Hebrew word yada is used five times. Can you find it anywhere? What is your yada relationship with God like? Write a prayer expressing your desire to be known and to know Him.*

Sexuality: A Sacred Picture

This may sound a little crazy, but sexuality is actually a physical picture of a deep spiritual truth. It's not just some random way God created us to have babies. The unrestrained passion, the vulnerability of being naked, the longing of unmet desire, the pleasure of sexual release, and the agony of betrayal all tell us a story . . . a story about God.

Let's break this down even further by looking at three specific and powerful ways sexuality is a holy metaphor—a sacred picture of God's love for us.

THE FREEDOM OF BEING KNOWN WITHIN THE SAFETY OF A COVENANT

We live in a world that views sex as a commodity to be traded. You trade your sexuality for companionship, reassurance of a man's love, or a fun night out. Because your sexuality is a commodity, you are constantly under evaluation and review. This means that if you don't please the person you are with, he will leave you. Unfortunately, this kind of thinking has permeated marriage. Couples "fall out of love" when one fails to please the other. You have to constantly perform, keep your figure, and please your man.

This was never how God intended sexuality to be expressed. Instead of a commodity to trade, it is a celebration of a promise. Only within a covenant (a promise that cannot be broken) are you free to be 100 percent who you are. You don't have to fear being naked, vulnerable, or rejected because the other person is never going away.

When sex is experienced within the safety of a true covenant, the pleasure and freedom is out of this world.

This is true of God's love for you. The Bible tells us that God loved us and gave His Son as a sacrifice while we were sinners with nothing to give back. You don't have to perform for God. Nothing you can do can separate you from His love if you have trusted Jesus as your Savior! He will never leave you nor forsake you!

THE AGONY OF BETRAYAL

Have you had a man promise to be faithful only to be betrayed? Have you witnessed the horrendous fallout of broken wedding vows between your parents? Few things rival the rejection of giving yourself fully to another person only to be discarded.

God knows this, which is why He says that sexuality should be reserved for the lifelong promise of marriage (Heb. 13:4). When God gave Himself to His people (Israel), they constantly chased after other gods. God used very sexual terms to describe their betrayal, calling them "prostitutes" and "adulterers" (Hos. 4:10–14).

The crushing pain of sexual infidelity and broken promises teaches us about God's jealousy for His people. Do you know that jealousy can be a good thing? The Bible says that God is a jealous God. In the same way, a married man should be "jealous" for his wife, and a wife "jealous" for her husband. My husband belongs to me. I don't want any other woman to see him naked or arouse him sexually. That is a holy jealousy, resembling God's heart that His people only worship Him. "You shall have no other gods before me" (Ex. 20:3 ESV).

THE LONGING OF SEPARATION

As a single woman, your sexuality may be represented by unending longings. You long to be close to someone—to give yourself fully. You daydream about what it will feel like to be face-to-face with a man you love and respect.

This longing also speaks of God's love. When Jesus was on the earth, He told His disciples that one day they would mourn and fast when He was taken away from them. He actually used the example of a bride waiting for the bridegroom to return. We may not fully understand this because our wedding traditions are different than the Jewish tradition Jesus was referring to. The process of getting married in ancient Jewish culture involved many stages. Right before the actual wedding, the bride knew that the groom would be coming soon but didn't know the exact hour. She had to wait and be ready for him whenever he surprised her. Jesus referred to this idea of being ready and waiting many times throughout His teaching.

The concept of waiting and longing is also in the Old Testament. The psalmists wrote about their deep yearnings and longings to be in God's presence. They weren't content to be separated from their Creator and God. "My heart and my flesh cry out for the living God. . . . As the deer pants for streams of water, so my soul pants for you, my God" (Ps. 84:2; 42:1).

Your sexuality paints a vivid, living picture of the gospel message. You were made for love, for deep knowing, and for the safety of a promise that can't be broken.

REFLECT AND RESPOND

- *What are some ways the world portrays sexuality as separate from the relational and spiritual aspects of yada? How has this impacted your thinking about sexuality?*

- *What do you think about the concept of your sexuality being connected with your relationship to God?*

- *Explain in your own words: how is sexuality a metaphor for intimacy with God? For your longing to know Him?*

Your Sexuality Cannot Be Separated from Your Spirituality

Here is perhaps the most profound truth I have learned by studying what God says about sex. Whether you are single or married, having great sex or no sex, your sexuality is inseparable from your spirituality.

Over and over again, you hear people suggest that sexual choices don't matter. Most of the people around you have bought into the lie that what you choose to do sexually is as trivial as what you had for breakfast. Sex is never just about sex. Our sexual opinions and choices ultimately reveal something much deeper about us and our relationship to God.

REFLECT AND RESPOND

- *Read 1 Corinthians 6:12–20 twice. The first time just read it all the way through. As you read it a second time, reflect on the text by answering the following questions:*

- *What is your body's purpose?*

- *What happens when two people come together?*

- *What one-word command are you given in regard to sexual immorality?*

- *What is unique about sexual sin in relation to every other sin?*

- *Ultimately, what does this passage say about the connection between who you are spiritually and who you are sexually?*

Our culture encourages you to explore sexually as a way of finding and expressing *who* you are. God wants you to think about your sexuality in terms of *whose* you are. Do you belong to God? Have you trusted in Him for life and salvation? If so, "you were bought with a price" (1 Cor. 6:20).

Research shows that you are more likely to make sexual decisions based on your generation than based on your profession of faith in God. Your opinions about living together before marriage, casual sex, LGBT issues, and pornography are more likely to reflect your age group and where you live than they are to reflect your belief in God.[1]

More important than your generational identity is your identity as God's daughter and a follower of Jesus Christ. Christians vary in age, race, experience, and geographical location, but our commitment to follow Jesus as Lord unites us.

Peter wrote it like this: "But you are a chosen people, a royal priesthood, a holy nation, God's special possession, that you may declare the praises of him who called you out of darkness into his wonderful light" (1 Peter 2:9). This is your "spiritual identity." How you think about and express your sexuality cannot be separated from that spiritual identity.

If you are like many Christian women, you have constructed a thick wall between your sexuality and your relationship with God. Your sexual desires and fantasies, your shame and temptations seem like a total disconnect from your longing to know and please God. Maybe it is your sexual thoughts that make you want to run away from God rather than run to Him. Your sexuality deeply impacts your spirituality and vice versa. Your confusion and hidden pain related to sex are inseparable from your relationship with God, even if you try compartmentalizing them. God cares about all of who you are, even the "sexual" you.

LIST 5 PHRASES THAT DESCRIBE YOUR SPIRITUAL IDENTITY: (1 PETER 2:9; 1 COR. 6:18–20)	LIST 5 WORDS THAT DESCRIBE WHAT YOU BELIEVE ABOUT YOUR SEXUALITY:
Example: I'm a temple of the Holy Spirit.	Example: My body is my own—I can do what I want with it.
1.	
2.	
3.	
4.	
5.	

Are your spiritual identity and your sexual beliefs consistent or at odds with each other?

For a long time, my view of God was so distorted. I never even looked at me being a sexual person and quenched all those desires somehow. And saying that, it wasn't that my thoughts were all pure. Sex/sexuality in my mind was not something to be addressed until after marriage. Yet when I'd hear men talking suggestively or referring to anything about sex or women, it infuriated me as a young lady.

It is in reading this I'm reminded that God loves us so much that He created us as sexual beings. When my view of God is so distorted, then I can't see sexuality as a gift from God. I only look at it as something I'm deprived of until marriage. I get so angry at the enemy for infiltrating lies! God really loves us. Our sexuality is a means of God inviting us to share those longings with Him. —Eve

REFLECT AND RESPOND

- *Like Eve, have you ever considered that your sexuality was meant to be an invitation to know the love of a Savior who will never reject you? Write a prayer to God asking Him to help you break down the thick wall between your sexuality and your relationship with Him.*

- *Today you read 1 Corinthians 6:19-20. If you are going to take this verse to heart, what needs to change?*

The Invitation

Ok, let's put it out there. Instead of being encouraged, you may just want to give up on this study. Hebrews 4:12 says that God's Word is like a two-edged sword, piercing our hearts. You may feel like the sword has been piercing you this week. The conviction of the Holy Spirit is different than feelings of guilt and condemnation. It's an invitation. While God's Word helps us recognize how we have rebelled against Him, the greater message of the Bible is an invitation to love and be loved. God is inviting you to trust Him with your sexuality, no matter how dirty, shameful, confused, or broken this area of your life may feel.

The greatest news in the Bible is summarized by this verse: "God demonstrates his own love for us in this: While we were still sinners, Christ died for us" (Rom. 5:8).

(Fill in the blanks with your own name, because this truth applies to you!)

God demonstrates His own love for _____ *in this: While*

_____ *was still a sinner, Christ died for* _____ !

God isn't waiting for you to get your sex life straightened out. He wants you to know His love, His forgiveness, and the freedom of living according to His plan for you. You don't have to have it all figured out; we are going to journey through this together over the next five weeks. The question is, Are you willing to say "yes" to His invitation to intimacy?

I feel like I have a head knowledge that God and marriage/sex is supposed to be an example of His love for me and the body of Christ, that Jesus is inviting us to be completely known by Him and vice versa; but I have no clue what that means personally. After being raped and having open sex with multiple partners, sex became something fun or something I had to do. I knew what I was doing wasn't as God designed, so I made it to be numbing and distanced myself even further from the Lord. I have asked and begged the Lord to show me what He really means sex to be in marriage and what He means in Scripture!

Now I'm realizing that our sexuality has a spiritual meaning! I sure hope it does. And I cannot wait to figure what all that entails and means! I know the Lord has such a complex, wonderful meaning of what it should be. I've seen in my life that I have searched in all the wrong places to be loved and known. I know that this is something the Lord has put deep inside all of us. Until the past six months or so I thought that would be found in a husband—I just had to keep waiting for this man to show up and fix everything. But having the recent jaw-dropping realization that I am not promised marriage made it even clearer that I have to be completely loved and satisfied in Jesus Christ. At that point, if the Lord decides to bring me a husband, great! But if not, that's okay because I will (hopefully) learn to become completely loved and known by the Father.
—Vanessa

REFLECT AND RESPOND

- *What would it look like for God to be the Lord of all of your life, including your sexuality?*

- *What barriers or fears are in the way of yielding this area of your life to God?*

- *Are some of your opinions of sexuality based on cultural norms and worldly desires? Make a list and pray for God to show you His truth on these things throughout the study.*

- *Write a prayer to God asking Him to tear down the barriers and fears through your time in this study.*
    (Example: "Jesus, I feel heavyhearted and a little confused. I know I have

been compartmentalizing my sexuality and have kept this piece of me away from You. Help me open up and understand what it means to invite You in and surrender my sexuality to You. Please free me from my guilt and shame and walk with me on this journey of understanding what it might look like to have a healthy sexuality.")

PULLING IT ALL TOGETHER

Below are key truths you have read about this week that also answer the questions posed at the start of the week. Now is the time to ask yourself, "How much have I embraced these truths in my life?" After each statement, circle the number (1-5) that represents the power of these truths in your life.

- Many parents and church leaders fail to teach a Christian view of sexuality.

    1   2   3   4   5

- God wants all of my life—even my sexuality—to be in agreement with His design for me.

    1   2   3   4   5

- I am sexual by God's design because He created me female, with the physical anatomy and biochemical properties of sexuality. I am still a sexual person whether or not I've had sex.

    1   2   3   4   5

- Sex, sexuality, and intimacy are often used interchangeably in our culture. My sexuality involves more than just having sex. The deeper purpose underneath my sexuality is the drive and desire to be known and loved.

  1   2   3   4   5

- I was made for intimacy with people but my greatest need for intimacy is to know the God who created me.

  1   2   3   4   5

- My sexuality is a holy metaphor of the gospel message. I was made for love, deep knowing, and for safety of a promise that can't be broken.

  1   2   3   4   5

- Many people's sexual choices are based on their generation's opinions rather than their spiritual identity.

  1   2   3   4   5

- How I think about and express my sexuality cannot be separated from my spiritual identity.

  1   2   3   4   5

- I need to accept God's invitation to trust Him with my sexuality. I don't have to get my sex life in order before saying yes to His invitation!

  1   2   3   4   5

Which truth did you rate the lowest? Write that truth on a 3x5 card (or on your phone) and look at it this week. Ask God to plant this truth in your heart.

Embracing

Have you ever asked yourself . . .

- *What modern opinion dismantled the foundational belief that I was created by a higher intelligent being?*
- *What is sexual atheism?*
- *What are the implications if I believe God designed my sexuality?*
- *Does God really expect me to control my sexual drive when the culture tells me otherwise?*
- *What is sexual integrity and how should it shape my daily choices?*
- *Besides being obedient to God's Word, what other reasons should motivate me to live with sexual integrity?*
- *Why do I still make foolish choices when I know better?*
- *What should I do if I've already messed up in the area of sexuality?*

This week's study, "Embracing a Grand Design," will bring you clarity on these questions and more. So let's get going!

a Grand
Design

You Are Sexual by Design

What do you think would happen to your body if you started training for a marathon? What if you cut out all sugar from your diet and began running several miles a day?

With some degree of confidence, you could predict changes like toned muscles, weight loss, increased stamina, and probably a few blisters along the way. Your body reacts to certain laws of science that make life semi-predictable. You can predict (or maybe you know from experience) how you will feel on three hours of sleep or after eating an entire container of ice cream.

Until the mid-1850s most of humanity agreed that we were created by some higher intelligent being. We explained the predictability of the sun and stars and of our own biology by attributing it to an intelligent Creator who designed the world with order. Then along came Darwin and the theory of evolution, which allowed for the possibility of human existence apart from a Creator. Much of our thinking about science, psychology, law, and morality has been dismantled by the modern belief that our existence is random, rather than determined by God.

How does this relate to sexuality? You have to decide between two worldviews. Either your sexuality was intentionally designed by your Creator or it has evolved as part of your humanity. If you embrace by faith that God created you, then you must accept that only He inherently has the authority to define sexual morality based on His design. If there is no creator, you have to figure out your own sexual ethics. Sexuality is either a random part of your humanity or it is an intentional aspect of God's design. Either God is God or you are on your own to figure out your existence. There truly is no middle ground.

Let me give you a practical example of what it means to live by faith and to accept God's authority over your life.

In 1999, John F. Kennedy Jr. and his wife died in a tragic plane crash off the coast of the Atlantic Ocean. The primary reason for the crash was that John was not "instrument rated" as a pilot. In other words, novice pilots navigate by what they see. Instrument-rated pilots have learned to fly by the instrument panel, even if the instruments seem to contradict what they perceive by looking out the window.

The National Transportation Safety Board concluded the cause of John's crash: "The pilot's failure to maintain control of the airplane during a descent over water at night, which was a result of spatial disorientation."[1] The weather obscured his vision and perception, and John thought he was flying much higher than he was. The instruments are not deceived by clouds or fog like human judgment can be. They determine altitude, air speed, and direction based on the laws of physics rather than perception. If John had trusted his instrument panel instead of his instincts, he would not have crashed.

Issues of sexuality can be confusing. The combination of your feelings, experiences, and the opinions of other people can swirl around you like a storm. Where do you look to find truth? You can choose to make decisions by "looking out of the window of the cockpit" or by trusting the "instrument panel" of God's Word.

When I am confused by what's around me or within me, I don't rely upon what I see or feel, but upon the God I worship. I know that God is close to the brokenhearted and compassionate in our struggles; I know that He is also righteous and holy.

I want to be an "instrument-rated" Christ follower, not swayed by the chaos of changing culture, but rooted in truths that are unchanging. What about you?

Legendary basketball coach John Wooden was a man who was instrument rated. Time and again, he referred to the tried and true principles of his Christian faith. Read this profound thought from Coach Wooden about living a life of integrity:

> Being true to ourselves doesn't make us people of integrity. Charles Manson was true to himself, and as a result, he rightly is spending the rest of his life in prison. Ultimately, being true to our Creator gives us the purest form of integrity.

In our humanistic culture, we have put as the highest good being "true to self." We are human centered, valuing life and individual identity as the greatest good. As Christians in a humanistic culture, we feel compelled to alter biblical teaching to support that goal. Scripture passages that seem to limit the full expression of a person are discounted as cultural or out of touch.

An instrument-rated Christian recognizes that life does and always has revolved around God rather than around human beings. "You are to be holy to me because I, the LORD, am holy" (Lev. 20:26). My desires, thoughts, and feelings are not the truest measure of who I am. My identity is rooted in my Creator—who God is—and my *choice* to worship Him.

Every day, you look around you and observe what is going on in this world. Perhaps you even look within yourself to discern how you think or feel. My question to you is this: Do you look regularly at the instrument panel of God's Word to be reminded of your Creator?

I meet many Christians who look to the instrument panel in many areas of their life, but think about their sexuality with a different approach. They want to honor God, but believe they can define their own sexual morality. Kenny Luck, founder of Every Man's Ministries, described a trend that he sees in Christian singles called sexual atheism. He says, "Practical sexual atheism among Christians means that God can speak into some things but not sex."[2]

We cannot say that Jesus is Lord of our lives but claim independence in our sexual thoughts and actions. If He is the Creator, than we must recognize the purpose of His design in all areas of life.

> I was a sexual atheist. I knew God created sex, but because I didn't understand the bigger picture, I didn't feel the need to submit that area of my life to Him. While it was easy to worship and obey Him in other areas of my life, I kept sexual sins and desires to myself. I think this was mostly due to guilt and shame. I knew God probably didn't approve of the decisions I was making, and frankly I didn't want to feel worse about myself. So I gave myself the freedom to make sexual decisions based on feelings, emotions, and desires, not knowing how this was so deeply tied to my spirituality. The more I tried to convince myself that I could be the "lord" of this area of my life, the further I felt from God. —Chelsey

REFLECT AND RESPOND

- *What are some evidences that many Christians (single and married) are "sexual atheists"?*

- *Are you a "sexual atheist" trying to find a middle ground? Why or why not?*

- *Do you think it is more difficult to submit your sexuality to God compared to other areas of your life? If so why?*

- *Last week, you read Psalm 139. Today, meditate on Psalm 139:13-16 specifically. Do you believe the statements David made are true about you? If so, what does this truth imply about your sexuality?*

God's Design Is for You to Live with Sexual Integrity

The hallmark of God's design for your sexuality is that it is meant to be integrated into the rest of your life. As mentioned in week 1, your sexuality is tied into who you are as a relational and spiritual woman.

God's design is for you to live with *sexual integrity*. Let's park there for a moment. The word *integrity* means "the state of being whole and undivided." To live with sexual integrity means that your sexuality is an outgrowth of the essence of who you are as a woman. When you live with sexual integrity, *your sexual choices are a consistent expression of your relational and spiritual commitments.*

Let's break that definition of sexual integrity down.

Sexual choices: Modern culture would have you believe that you don't have sexual choices. In essence, they teach that you are animalistic and driven by hormones and irresistible urges. The Bible distinguishes human beings from all creation in that we have moral choices in all areas, including how to express our sexuality. Only humans were created in God's image with the moral capacity and responsibility to choose good and evil. After God created the world, the animals, fish of the sea, and birds of the air, He created the man and woman, blessed them, and charged them to: "Be fruitful and increase in number; fill the earth and subdue it. Rule over the fish in the sea and the birds in the sky and over every living creature that moves on the ground" (Gen. 1:28). He gave Adam and Eve the opportunity to obey or disobey His divine authority. We still have the freedom to choose to honor God or to reject His authority in every area of life, including our sexuality.

Consistent expression: You make choices about your sexuality every day—what to look at, what to think about, how much of your heart and body to give away, and how to deal with your sexual past.

PULLING IT ALL TOGETHER

Take a few minutes now and reflect on each of these sexual choices. Use the scale to score yourself.

1 = The choice I make in this area of my life is under my personal control.

10 = The choice I make in this area of my life is surrendered to God.

What I look at:

1   2   3   4   5   6   7   8   9   10

What I think about:

1   2   3   4   5   6   7   8   9   10

How much of my heart and body I give away:

1   2   3   4   5   6   7   8   9   10

How I deal with my sexual past:

1   2   3   4   5   6   7   8   9   10

Relational and spiritual commitments: Your Creator's intention is for your sexuality to be consistent with your relational and spiritual commitments. The hallmark of broken sexuality is when our sexual actions are completely separate from the promises we've made to other people and God.

• *What promises does a woman make when she gets married?*

• *What promises does a woman make when she accepts Christ into her life?*

Broken sexuality is expressed by single *and* married women when their sexual choices don't match their *relational commitments*. Let me explain . . .

A *single woman with broken sexuality*:
If you sleep with a guy you are dating you lack sexual integrity. You are celebrating with your bodies what you have not chosen to do with your whole lives within the promise of marriage. My husband, Mike, and I pledged on our wedding day to be devoted to each other and to live life with a united purpose. Every time we have sex, we are remembering and celebrating the spiritual and relational commitment we made to each other.

A *married woman with broken sexuality*:
If I chose to have sex with a man other than my husband, I would be violating not just my wedding vows, but my life would lack integrity. My sexual choices would be totally inconsistent with my desire to love God and my promise to love my husband. I would also lack sexual integrity if I stopped having sex with my husband. My sexuality should be a consistent expression of my commitment to Mike. Perhaps this is why Paul told married couples to be sexually intimate on a regular basis (see 1 Cor. 7:1–5).

Broken sexuality is expressed by single *and* married women when their sexual choices don't match their *spiritual commitment* to follow the Lord. If Jesus is her Savior, her body (including her sexuality) no longer belongs to her but should be used for God's glory. As a follower of Christ, she cannot pick and choose which areas to surrender to God. Either He is the Lord of her life or He's not.

This is so critical, that I'd like you to take time right now to personally evaluate your own sexual integrity.

• *What have you promised to God?*

____ *I have professed Jesus Christ as my Lord and Savior. (When and where did this take place? What was your age and the circumstances that led up to it?)*

____ *I have not professed Jesus Christ as my Lord and Savior. (What is holding you back? List any negative experiences or lingering questions that keep you from making a commitment to Christ.)*

• *What have you promised to a man?*
____ *I have committed my life to a man who is my husband through marriage.*

____ *I have not committed my life to a man through marriage yet. (List your current relationship status: _____ (example: single, dating, seriously dating, engaged, divorced).*

• *If someone were to look at your choices, what would they conclude about you as a person?*

• *Are your sexual actions consistent with your relational and spiritual commitments? Why or why not?*

- *If your choices are not consistent, what needs to change? What is one thing you can do today in pursuit of sexual integrity? (Check out James 1:22–25.)*

- *In your own words, write a definition of sexual integrity.*

- *Here is Juli's summary of God's design for sexuality: "God's design is for your sexual choices to accurately reflect your devotion to Him and to reveal the level of commitment you've made to a man." Write your own summary below.*

The Wisdom Principle

One of my greatest joys as a Christian psychologist is seeing how what the Bible teaches actually lines up with what is best for us. The book of Proverbs says that God made the world (including human beings) with wisdom woven into the very fabric of His creation. In the following passage of Proverbs, wisdom is speaking:

"The LORD brought me forth as the first of his works,
  before his deeds of old;
I was formed long ages ago,
  at the very beginning, when the world came to be.
When there were no watery depths, I was given birth,
  when there were no springs overflowing with water;
before the mountains were settled in place,
  before the hills, I was given birth,
before he made the world or its fields
  or any of the dust of the earth.
I was there when he set the heavens in place,
  when he marked out the horizon on the face of the deep,
when he established the clouds above
  and fixed securely the fountains of the deep,
when he gave the sea its boundary
  so the waters would not overstep his command,
and when he marked out the foundations of the earth.
  Then I was constantly at his side.
I was filled with delight day after day,

rejoicing always in his presence,
rejoicing in his whole world
and delighting in mankind." (Prov. 8:22–31)

I like to bake special treats for my family. Flour is one of the primary ingredients I use when baking. Cookies, pies, muffins . . . they all have flour. Before something goes in the oven, I blend all of the other ingredients with the flour so that flour becomes absolutely absorbed into the eggs, sugar, and everything else. Try taking the flour out of a chocolate chip cookie after it is baked. It's impossible. What this passage teaches is that God's wisdom was "baked" into every aspect of creation. You can never extract His wisdom from the earth, the skies, the ocean, animals, or human beings. When you study them, you study wisdom.

This is why when we study anything from gravity to animal behavior, we see predictable laws that bring order to the world. God created the world *with wisdom*, giving order and purpose to all He made.

The entire book of Proverbs is a father pleading for his son to study wisdom and to follow the design of God's creation. He tells his son to study the wisdom of everything from how ants work to the foolishness of a beautiful woman who has no discretion. Solomon (who wrote most of the proverbs) talks about two different kinds of people: wise people who live according to God's authority and design and foolish people who ignore God's authority and design.

God created your mind, body, and soul with principles of His wisdom that you can never escape. You can ignore them, but you can't be free from them. Just like the laws of gravity govern what happens when you jump off a building, the moral principles of wisdom dictate what happens when we make foolish sexual and relational choices.

REFLECT AND RESPOND

• *Read Proverbs 1:7. What does this verse say about the difference between the wise person and foolish person?*

• *How can stepping outside of God's design be destructive?*

Social science research is filled with examples of how a lack of sexual integrity (living outside of God's design) is physically and emotionally destructive. Here are a few of them:

PORNOGRAPHY

Research overwhelmingly demonstrates that watching pornography (or reading erotic material) diminishes sexual fulfillment over time. Although it may immediately heighten the experience of arousal, it actually makes your partner (or future partner) less sexually fulfilling. Pornography trains your brain to respond to unrealistic sexual images and allows you to have a sexual experience on your own terms. The long-term effect? A man or woman cannot respond sexually within a real relationship that requires patience, understanding, and communication. In fact, research is now linking porn use to erectile dysfunction among young men.[3]

• *How do porn and erotica distort the way God's design was meant to function in real relationships?*

COHABITATION

While modern wisdom promotes living together before or instead of marriage, research consistently says that this is a bad idea. Couples living together are more likely to experience sexual unfaithfulness, domestic violence, and divorce if they eventually do get married. Why? Living together fosters a consumer mentality toward sexuality and relationship. You are "on trial," testing each other out. If at any point the relationship isn't meeting your needs or his, you can bail.

Even if a couple decides to get married after cohabiting, this attitude of "squishy" commitment may follow them into marriage. Waiting to live together until marriage fosters a completely different tone in the relationship. The vows "till death do us part," mean that you are committing to each other no matter what. You are promising to love and be faithful even when you disappoint each other. God says not to give yourself fully to someone outside of this covenant love. Why? Because you are not a consumer product. Your sexuality wasn't designed to be bartered and traded, but to be a celebration of unconditional love and acceptance.

• *Why do you think the culture has so wholeheartedly approved of living together?*

SAFE SEX

Health organizations that used to teach us to have "safe sex" by wearing a condom or taking birth control have changed their language to encourage "safer sex." They've had to acknowledge that any sexual encounter, including oral sex, puts you at risk for STDs. The only absolutely safe way to have sex is for two virgins to have sex only with each other for their entire lives. Wait . . . that sounds like God's design for marriage!

> Sex before marriage damaged my views on God's design of sexuality because there was no stability or commitment and everything felt chaotic. Although it may have been fun for a moment, that was always fleeting. I turned it into a game of control to get what I wanted and I tried to fill a void that was searching for acceptance, affirmation, and love, but it always left me feeling emptier than before. It was the most numbing and shameful thing I have ever experienced.
> —Ally

What the Bible says about sexuality isn't some stuffy, out-of-date religious teaching. It reflects how the Designer created you to thrive. Sexual integrity isn't just about honoring God, it is also what is best for you.

God's design for sexuality is literally written on your body and wired into your moral fiber. When sexuality is expressed within the parameters of that design (marriage), we see the impact of great blessings.

THE ROLE OF OXYTOCIN IN MARRIAGE

When a couple is regularly sexually active, important chemicals including dopamine (the feel-good hormone) and endorphins (which relieves stress) are released. One of the most important hormones to be released is oxytocin. Oxytocin has been nicknamed "the cuddle hormone" because of its role in bonding. Mothers get huge amounts of oxytocin when they give birth or breast-feed. This causes the mom to fall in love with her newborn. When a married couple gets regular doses of oxytocin through sexual intimacy, their brains are being wired to bond with one another over and over again.

As much as our society wants to pretend that God's design doesn't matter, the above empirical research (and more not listed) continues to show us that it does.

REFLECT AND RESPOND

- *Read Proverbs 6:23-33. What does the father warn his son about in this passage?*

- *The warning is the same for women. What does the Bible say happens if or when you step outside of God's design for sex?*

- *Read Proverbs 5:18-19. This same father encourages his son where to find sexual pleasure. How can sex be a blessing within marriage?*

The Folly Principle

Yesterday, we looked at God's wisdom—how it is integrated into creation and how wise people study and apply God's design to every part of their lives. We looked at how living by wisdom keeps us from harm and leads to God's blessing. Pretty simple concept, right? Unfortunately, most of us don't live by principles of wisdom. The average intelligent, educated, Christian woman makes choices that fly in the face of wisdom—particularly related to her sexuality.

Growing up I was very promiscuous. I was never sexually abused or anything like that. I actually had a wonderful, healthy, and happy childhood. In Pre-K I was kissing boys and going inside the bathroom with them to see their penis. I don't remember exactly when this started, but I used to play house with another girl and we started kissing because I was playing mom and she was playing dad. Unfortunately after a while we just got in a room and kissed all the time. Thankfully I am not attracted to women. I kept kissing boys in school all the time, but never had sex of any kind.

During my freshman year of college, I gave into the pressure and had sex with an old high school boyfriend. We didn't start dating or anything; I literally just called him for sex. After being with him, I started sleeping around. I had sex with about fifteen guys in about a year. Then I fell in love with a guy, so we started living together. I got pregnant in 2003 and then again in 2004. After the second abortion I tried to commit suicide, and that's when the Lord showed up in my life.

With the help of the Holy Spirit I was able to retrain/reprogram my mind. I learned not to flirt or be sexually active with every man that crossed my path. At the beginning of this process I couldn't be around men. I couldn't even look them in the eye.

I am very passionate and enjoyed sex a lot back in the day. It was hard, actually extremely hard, for me to stay pure. I was pure from 2004 until 2012. In November 2012 I rebelled against God and started having sex again with my boyfriend at the time. Ironically (or by the grace of God) I could not enjoy it. I couldn't have an orgasm, I couldn't give myself completely or be completely present, I didn't have the "power" I used to have over a man during sex. I was extremely miserable throughout the entire sexual experience. I believe it was because of the Holy Spirit in me. Also I was in disobedience, outside of His will. I haven't had sex since February 2013. It is actually a miracle that I am not sleeping around. I pray hard for protection and for God to help me stay pure until my wedding night. —Morgan

Morgan's testimony presents a picture of how we desire to live by wisdom but end up making foolish choices. One bad choice can lead to another, then another until we feel trapped. God intervened in Morgan's life. He offers each one of us forgiveness, redemption, and a chance to start over.

Paul quoted Old Testament writers in his letter to the Roman church, "There is no one righteous, not even one; there is no one who understands; there is no one who seeks God. All have turned away, they have together become worthless; there is no one who does good, not even one" (Rom. 3:10–12).

Every single one of us has a rebellious, foolish heart. We think we know better than God does. Only by the work of His love within us do we worship and seek Him.

Your sexual choices and attitudes represent a continual battlefield, pitting wisdom against folly and God's authority against your desire to run your own life. In tomorrow's study, you will read about how to ask God to help you live in His wisdom and forgiveness!

REFLECT AND RESPOND

- *Proverbs illustrates this battle with "voices" that call out to us. Read Proverbs 1:20–33.*

• *What does wisdom cry out to people?*

• *Verse 22 lists three different kinds of people who don't listen to wisdom. How would you describe the "simple," the "mocker," and the "fool"?*

• *What happens to a person who constantly rejects wisdom? Have you seen this happen to people you know?*

• *When you think about your sexual choices and attitudes, do they reflect wisdom? Why or why not?*

• *Read Proverbs 1:23. What does wisdom (God) promise when you repent of your rebellion and folly?*

Jesus Offers You a Way Forward

How do you feel as you read about God's design for sexuality? Maybe it gives you hope and strengthens your resolve to follow Him. But maybe this information has heaped guilt on your shoulders because God's truth is shining a light into a dark corner of your life. Write your feelings in the space below:

_____

_____

_____

_____

_____

_____

_____

Women often ask me what they should do if they've already messed up in the area of sexuality. Is it possible to go back? While we can't go back and erase the choices we've made, Jesus offers us a way forward. Every single follower of Christ was once a foolish, rebellious sinner. Every pastor, every missionary, every disciple would say with John Newton, "I once was lost, but now am found, was blind, but now I see!"

Yielding your sexuality to the Creator's design is not just about being sexually pure. Jesus also came to redeem us in our sin and heal our brokenness. You may have a tangled mess of sin and sexual trauma in your past. You know firsthand how devastating sexuality can be when it is outside of God's design. Your Creator invites you to healing and redemption. This study is designed to help you on that journey.

When Jesus began His ministry, He referenced a prophecy from the book of Isaiah and basically said, "This is why I am here": "The Spirit of the Lord is on me, because he has anointed me to proclaim good news to the poor. He has sent me to proclaim freedom for the prisoners and recovery of sight to the blind, to set the oppressed free, to proclaim the year of the Lord's favor" (Luke 4:18–19).

God's design is for you to be free—free from sin, condemnation, shame, and bondage! Because of decisions you have made, you may feel like "damaged goods," but God does not see you that way. He loves you and longs to redeem your life. Nothing is beyond His healing and forgiveness!

Living with sexual integrity also applies to how you now respond to the choices you have made in the past. Do you believe that Jesus died to forgive you and free you from sin? Second Corinthians 5:17 says, "Therefore, if anyone is in Christ, the new creation has come: The old has gone, the new is here!" If you are in Christ, living with integrity means that God has made all things new. Will you ask Him to make this a reality in your heart today?

You can't move forward in wholeness without dealing with your past. Our enemy, Satan, loves for us to believe that we are defined by the past, that forgiveness may be for heaven, but we can't ever be free from our choices here on earth. God has given us a specific way to be cleansed and free from our past. It's called confession.

David, who committed adultery and murder, wrote about the difference between hiding his sin and confessing it to God:

Oh, what joy for those whose disobedience is forgiven, whose sin is put out of sight! Yes, what joy for those whose record the Lord has cleared of guilt, whose lives are lived in complete honesty! When I refused to confess my sin, my body wasted away, and I groaned all day long. Day and night your hand of discipline was heavy on me. My strength evaporated like water in the summer heat. Finally, I confessed all my sins to you and stopped trying to hide my guilt. I said to myself, "I will confess my rebellion to the Lord." And you forgave me! All my guilt is gone. (Ps. 32:1–5 NLT)

REFLECT AND RESPOND

• *Describe how David felt when he hid his sin. Now describe how he felt after confessing his sin.*

• *Do you feel more like David felt before he confessed or after?*

• *Is there something specific you need to confess to the Lord? If so, what's holding you back?*

• *Write a prayer expressing what you've learned this week and specifically how you believe God wants to set you free.*

PULLING IT ALL TOGETHER

Below are key truths you have read about this week that also answer the questions posed at the start of the week. Now is the time to ask yourself, "How much have I embraced this truth in my life?" After each statement, circle the number (1–5) that represents the power of this truth in your life.

• Sexual atheism is when Christians give God authority over some areas of their life but not their sex life.

1   2   3   4   5

- I cannot say that Jesus is Lord of my life. I choose my own sexual ethics.

1   2   3   4   5

- The culture teaches that my sexual drive is beyond my control and driven by hormones. The Bible distinguishes human beings from all creation in that we have moral choices in all areas, including sexuality.

1   2   3   4   5

- Sexual integrity = God's design is for my sexual choices to accurately reflect my devotion to Him and to reveal the level of commitment I've made to a man.

1   2   3   4   5

- If Jesus is my Savior, my body no longer belongs to me but should be used for God's glory.

1   2   3   4   5

- God created my mind, body, and soul with principles of His wisdom that I can never escape. I can ignore them, but I can't be free from them.

1   2   3   4   5

- Sexual integrity isn't just about honoring God, it's also what is best for me.

1   2   3   4   5

- Every single one of us has a rebellious, foolish heart and only by the work of His love do we seek Him.

1   2   3   4   5

- My sexual choices and attitudes represent a continual battlefield, pitting wisdom against folly and God's authority against my desire to run my own life.

  1   2   3   4   5

- While I can't go back and erase the choices I've made, Jesus offers me a way forward.

  1   2   3   4   5

- Beyond being sexually pure, God designed me to be free from sin, condemnation, shame, and bondage.

  1   2   3   4   5

- To move forward in my newfound freedom, I must believe God has restored me. I am new!

  1   2   3   4   5

Which truth did you rate the lowest? Write that truth on a 3x5 card (or on your phone) and look at it this week. Ask God to plant this truth in your heart.

Sexuality Your

Have you ever asked yourself . . .

- *Do I believe God's intentions for me are good?*
- *What do I want most out of life, happiness or holiness?*
- *What is God's purpose in allowing me to face sexual struggles?*
- *What is worship? And how is sexual integrity an act of worship?*

This week's study, "Sexuality and Your Character," will bring you clarity on these questions and more. So let's jump in!

and

Character

God Cares about Your Character

During my four years in college, I played competitive tennis. Now, I look back at all of the hours I spent training and practicing and wonder if it was worth it. Back then, winning or losing a match was everything, but a few decades have put things into perspective. Still, I'm glad I played tennis, not because of how many matches I won, but because of the lessons I learned.

Hobbies like sports and music are great tools for developing character. You learn to work as a team, how to push through the discomfort of training, and how to handle both success and failure. My time playing tennis helped me develop into the person I am today. God used the experience of a team sport to teach me important life disciplines that carry over into adult life.

I believe your sexuality is very similar. Some single women wonder, "Why do I have these sexual feelings and urges if I can't act on them? What's the point?" Perhaps more than any other area of your life, your sexuality can be a powerful tool through which the Lord tests and refines your character, making you more like Him. This is not only true for single women. God has used the sexual struggles in my marriage to reveal and test my character more than any other area of marriage. Throughout more than twenty years of marriage, I've had to learn to be understanding, unselfish, forgiving, merciful, and courageous in overcoming fear. I can't think of any area of marriage that has challenged me more than the sexual aspect.

As we discussed in week 1, many Christian women have learned to separate their sexuality from the other areas of life. Sexuality is sometimes seen as dirty, shameful, and purely physical while spirituality is lofty, holy, and honorable. One thing I hope you learn from this study is that the wall between your sexuality and your spirituality is imaginary. Your sexual choices *are* spiritual choices. God cares about your sexuality because it unveils your heart. How you respond to your sexual desires and wounds tells a lot about your character. Sexuality is a realistic, tangible testing ground. We can sing to God at church and tell people how much we love Him, but the truth is revealed through how we live.

Let's look at a couple of events recorded in the Bible to illustrate the connection between sexuality and character.

JOSEPH

You probably know at least a little about Joseph's life. He was the favorite son of his father, Jacob, and his brothers had it in for him so they sold him to slave traders (now that's sibling rivalry!). Joseph ends up in the house of a ruler named Potiphar. He does such a great job that he is promoted to becoming Potiphar's right-hand man. We will pick up Joseph's story in Genesis 39:

Now Joseph was handsome in form and appearance. And after a time his master's wife cast her eyes on Joseph and said, "Lie with me." But he refused and said to his master's wife, "Behold, because of me my master has no concern about anything in the house, and he has put everything that he has in my charge. He is not greater in this house than I am, nor has he kept back anything from me except you, because you are his wife. How then can I do this great wickedness and sin against God?" And as she spoke to Joseph day after day, he would not listen to her, to lie beside her or to be with her.

But one day, when he went into the house to do his work and none of the men of the house was there in the house, she caught him by his garment, saying, "Lie with me." But he left his garment in her hand and fled and got out of the house. And as soon as she saw that he had left his garment in her hand and had fled out of the house, she called to the men of her household and said to them, "See, he has brought among us a Hebrew to laugh at us. He came in to me to lie with me, and I cried out with a loud voice. And as soon as he heard that I lifted up my voice and cried out, he left his garment beside me and fled and got out of the house." Then she laid up his garment by her until his master came home, and she told him the same story, saying, "The Hebrew servant, whom you have brought among us, came in to me to laugh at me. But as soon as I lifted up my voice and cried, he left his garment beside me and fled out of the house." (Gen. 39:6–18 ESV)

REFLECT AND RESPOND

• *How did this episode in Joseph's life test his character?*

• *What did you learn about Joseph through how he reacted to the temptation?*

• *What did you learn about the character of Potiphar's wife?*

SAMSON

Remember this guy? He was set apart from birth to be a leader of the Israelites. For all of his strengths, Samson had some serious character flaws that were revealed through his sexuality.

REFLECT AND RESPOND

• *Read the following snapshots from Samson's life: Judges 14:1–3 and 16:1–21.*

• *Do you think Samson saw any connection between his call to serve God and his sexual choices? Why or why not?*

• *What did you learn about Samson's character through the ways he approached his sexuality?*

• *How may God be using your sexuality to test your character?*

• *What do your sexual choices and beliefs reveal about your character?*

• *Why do you think God might use sexuality to refine and reveal your character?*

Sexuality and Worship

Behind your sexuality is a greater spiritual battle, prompting you to ask three important questions: Who do I worship? Is God really good? What is God's purpose for my life?

This week, we will take each one individually and consider why it's an important question to be asking.

1. WHO DO I WORSHIP?

Paul wrote a letter to the Roman church that became the book of Romans in our modern Bibles. The Roman culture was characterized by sexual, moral, and relational chaos. Take a moment to read Paul's description in Romans 1:

> We see the anger of God coming down from heaven against all the sins of men. These sinful men keep the truth from being known. Men know about God. He has made it plain to them. Men cannot say they do not know about God. From the beginning of the world, men could see what God is like through the things He has made. This shows His power that lasts forever. It shows that He is God. They did know God, but they did not honor Him as God. They were not thankful to Him and thought only of foolish things. Their foolish minds became dark. They said that they were wise, but they showed how foolish they were. They gave honor to false gods that looked like people who can die and to birds and animals and snakes. This honor belongs to God who can never die.
>
> So God let them follow the desires of their sinful hearts. They did sinful things among themselves with their bodies. They traded the truth of God for a lie. They worshiped and cared for what God made instead of worshiping the God Who made it. He is the One Who is to receive honor and thanks forever. Let it be so.

Because of this, God let them follow their sinful desires, which lead to shame. Women used their bodies in ways God had not planned. In the same way, men left the right use of women's bodies. They did sex sins with other men. They received for themselves the punishment that was coming to them for their sin.

Because they would not keep God in their thoughts anymore, He gave them up. Their minds were sinful and they wanted only to do things they should not do. They are full of everything that is sinful and want things that belong to others. They hate people and are jealous. They kill other people. They fight and lie. They do not like other people and talk against them. They talk about people, and they hate God. They are filled with pride and tell of all the good they do. They think of new ways to sin. They do not obey their parents. They are not able to understand. They do not do what they say they will do. They have no love and no loving-pity. They know God has said that all who do such things should die. But they keep on doing these things and are happy when others do them also. (Rom. 1:18–32 NLT)

Paul's discussion about homosexuality typically gets the most attention when we read this passage. However, this passage is not first and foremost about sex, it is actually about worship. This pagan culture began their moral decline when they dethroned God as the Creator who is to be worshiped.

Read the passage again and notice that before Paul even talks about sexual and other immoral choices, he teaches about the tragedy of people refusing to worship God.

REFLECT AND RESPOND

- *Circle two or three choices the Romans made in their worship according to Romans 1:18–27.*

- *Underline five results their godless worship had on society's morality and sexual behavior (Rom. 1:28–32).*

• How do you see this same pattern playing out in your world and in our churches today?

In Paul's day, rebellion against God looked like idol worship. The Greek and Roman cultures had many gods, most of them connected to nature. When you read Paul's letter to the Romans, it seems silly to worship statues of "animals and snakes." But in our modern culture, we have our own form of idol worship. We worship the intellect by elevating science above everything and we worship humanity by defining truth primarily based on how we think and feel.

In today's humanistic culture, we have elevated the experience of self. "Look inside yourself. Be true to yourself!" This is absolutely terrible advice. If I lived by it, I would love my husband one day and want to kill him the next. I would feel secure in my femininity for a season and then doubt myself through another season. There is also a danger in defining truth by the latest "wisdom." Over the past twenty years, our culture has done a complete 180 in defining sexual morality and health. What was called sinful and dysfunctional just a short time ago, is now celebrated as a worthy lifestyle.

When we make decisions about what we believe (about sexuality or anything) we begin with a compass that helps us define truth. The source you rely upon for your foundation of truth reveals your god. If you look "inward" for truth, you worship self. If you look "outward" for truth, you worship other people or rationalism. If you look "upward" for truth, you worship God.

While Romans 1 describes an entire culture, the same pattern can play out in each of our individual lives. We each face a lot of pressure in today's culture to reject God's design for sexuality. Even among Christians today, God's truth has taken a backseat to each person's right to pursue his or her own sexual fulfillment and create his or her own sexual morality. When we reject God as the *only* One with the authority to determine morality, we begin to compromise and make moral choices based on what "feels right." The choices you make about your sexuality begin by answering the question, Who do I worship?

REFLECT AND RESPOND

When do you find yourself looking:

"inward"? _____

"outward"? _____

"upward"? _____

Do you believe that God is the Sovereign Lord and that only He has the authority to determine right and wrong? *God's truth will at times fly in the face of what you feel and experience.* This is why faith actually requires faith (go figure!) to believe a truth that momentarily seems very untrue. It is a lot easier to live according to the world's mantra giving each person the right to define truth for herself. This is not only a question for single women. Sexual purity is a battle for men and women of all ages and marital status. It means saying to God, "I want to honor You in my sexuality, no matter how that looks in this stage of my life." It takes faith and courage to hold to a standard of truth the world hates. But that, my friend, is worship.

REFLECT AND RESPOND

• *In your own words, describe the meaning of worship.*

• *If someone were to look at only your sexuality and the sexual choices you make (including your thought life), would they conclude that your life is submitted to worshiping God?*

• *How is sexual integrity an act of worship?*

• *What needs to change in your life for God to be worshiped in your sexuality?*

When I first asked myself this question—"If someone were to look at only your sexuality and the sexual choices you make (including your thought life), would they conclude that your life is submitted to worshiping God?"—I was hit by a wave of shame. I felt like Eve in the garden—suddenly naked and exposed. I had always assumed my thought life was my own, my private property and my own problem. The idea that my thoughts were part of my worship to God was new and transformative. —Chelsey

2. Is God Really Good?

Sexuality has put God on trial. I don't think that's too strong of a statement! God's love and kindness have come under scrutiny because His Word appears to be keeping people from happiness and fulfillment. Here are some common statements that I hear (and I'm pretty sure you've heard or even had similar thoughts):

"A loving God would never give someone sexual desires and then tell her she can't fulfill them!"

"God understands that I'm lonely. He hasn't brought marriage, but He must be okay with me having sex or reading erotica. What does He expect me to do?"

"All God cares about is love, whether that love is expressed in a homosexual relationship or heterosexual, in marriage or living together."

God, in His goodness, calls us to live with self-control (see Heb. 13:4; 1 Cor. 6:18–20; 1 Thess. 4:3–8). God tells us *not* to satisfy every desire we feel. For some people, this makes God seem like an old-fashioned, uncaring tyrant. I've had many women respond to clear biblical teaching on sexuality by saying, "Well, that's not the God I serve!" They just can't accept that a loving God would ever say "no" to our desire to express our sexuality the way we want to.

Is this true of you?

1   2   3   4   5   6   7   8   9   10

(1 = not true of you at all, 10 = completely true of you)

Satan has always aimed primarily at getting people to doubt the goodness of God. Oswald Chambers claimed that all sin is rooted in the suspicion that God is not really good—that He is holding out on us.[1] This was the objective of the first lie—the first temptation—in the garden of Eden. He convinced Eve that God was keeping her from something good and she believed him!

REFLECT AND RESPOND

• *Read Genesis 3:1-7. How was Satan's lie an attack on God's character? Why do you think Eve believed Satan?*

• *How does a worldly perspective on sex make you think that God is keeping you from something good?*

• *How does Satan use your sexuality to tempt you to doubt God's character?*

If you take God's design for sex seriously, that will mean saying "no" to a lot of things you may want. It might mean saying "no" to dating a guy who wants to have sex with you. It means saying "no" when all of your friends are going to the latest sexually explicit movie. It means saying "no" to the sexual expression your body may be craving in the moment. These examples of self-denial might make you wonder why God would want you to feel dissatisfied and uncomfortable.

Hebrews 11:6 says, "Without faith it is impossible to please God, because anyone who comes to him must believe that he exists and that he rewards those who earnestly seek him." It takes faith to trust the goodness of God when His commands cause you discomfort. Only by faith will you believe that God's call for your temporary discomfort and self-denial serves an eternal purpose. Living according to God's design at times *will* cause pain and disruption.

I want to clarify that this does not mean that sexual desire is evil or shameful. It means that we submit those desires (and all desires) to God's will for our lives. This is what Jesus meant when He said, "Whoever wants to be my disciple must deny themselves and take up their cross daily and follow me" (Luke 9:23). Walking by faith, we believe that the goodness of God calls us to rewards greater than the temporary pleasure of getting what we want right now.

The rewards of a godly life may not be Prince Charming waiting in the wings or happily ever after in marriage. Sometimes God brings those gifts, but He never promised them. The spiritual blessings God gives His disciples are hard to see but impossible to deny. The apostle Peter described it this way, "Though you have not seen him, you love him; and even though you do not see him now, you believe in him and are filled with an inexpressible and glorious joy" (1 Peter 1:8).

Earlier in the week, we looked at a snapshot in Joseph's life. This young man must have doubted the goodness of God when he was sold into slavery and then falsely accused and punished for making the "right" choice! God's goodness in Joseph's life was played out in a dramatic way that took many years to unfold. The Lord fulfilled the dreams and promises He had given to Joseph as a young boy. Even though your story isn't likely to be as dramatic as Joseph's, your God is the same God that redeemed Joseph's life and blessed his obedience.

No one can promise you what God's blessings for faithfulness and obedience will look like. But God is good. He is for you. Honoring His Word and trusting Him are worth it!

REFLECT AND RESPOND

- *Read John 10:10. What are Satan's intentions for your life?*

- *What are Jesus' intentions for your life?*

- *Do you trust that God's design for intimacy is the best for you right now? Why or why not?*

I'd been speaking to teens on sexuality for over a decade and living with sexual integrity as a single woman myself. I loved what I did for a living yet deeply desired to be married and have children. With each passing birthday, I began to wonder if God would bring me a "holy hunk." I knew He didn't owe it to me but I was determined to remain hopeful.

While deeply entrenched in my speaking career, I was asked to do a radio interview to advertise one of my upcoming speaking events. Greg heard the interview and decided to attend the event just to meet me. During the first couple minutes of the event, I noticed Greg in the audience and found myself completely distracted. It was as if a spotlight fell on him and no one else was in the room. It sounds cheesy but it's the truth! (I thought, "He's probably married to a fabulous woman and she's at home with their three kids. Focus, Abby. Focus!") I regained concentration and delivered a strong message to the group in attendance. Afterward, I was pleasantly surprised when Greg courageously made his way to the front of the room and introduced himself. It quickly became evident he wasn't married with three kids back home! We hit it off and began dating. Six months later, we were engaged and shortly after my 35th birthday, I married my "holy hunk"! A lot can change in a short period of time. A season of life that felt like it would never end came to a close in a matter of a moment. —Abby

My boyfriend and I moved to a new city at the same time. We were recent college grads and flat broke. It would have been way easier to find a place and move in together. All of our friends recommended it and family members even suggested it would be a way to save money. Of course we wanted to live together, but we knew what this could lead to and wanted to honor God with our relationship. We got separate apartments and found extra work to pay the bills. It was hard. We got made fun of. But we protected our relationship that later ended in marriage. Honoring God's design is not easy, but we were able to experience firsthand how He blesses obedience. —Erin

Sex and God's Plan for You

3. WHAT IS GOD'S PURPOSE FOR YOUR LIFE?

It can be easy to forget that God has a greater goal than your personal happiness. His plans for your life are beyond anything this world can compete with. Romans 8:28 is one of the most encouraging and popular verses in the Bible: "And we know that in all things God works for the good of those who love him, who have been called according to his purpose."

What is His purpose? You have to keep reading through to the next verse . . . "For God knew his people in advance, and he chose them to become like his Son, so that his Son would be the firstborn among many brothers and sisters" (Rom. 8:29 NLT).

God's purpose for your life is that you would become a spiritual daughter, becoming like Jesus in your heart and character. What if your sexuality is one of the primary ways God achieves this goal in your life? What if He chose sexuality as a real-life learning lab to teach you Christlike character traits like humility, self-control, kindness, and forgiveness?

My guess is that it costs you something right now to follow Jesus. As you learned in day 3, there are things you desire that you say "no" to because you want to honor the Lord. That is normal and part of how God will transform your character to become more like His. Think about the way Jesus lived on earth. We see over and over again that He refused to follow His own wisdom and desires, but submitted to doing the will of His Father. God wants to develop that kind of character in you and me. He just might use sexuality as the testing ground to accomplish this holy purpose.

• *Read 2 Corinthians 12:7–10. How did God use Paul's struggle to make him more like Christ?*

• *How is God using the area of sexuality to make you more like Him?*

I've heard many Christians say that their goal is to "save themselves for marriage." While this is a wonderful goal, it is not the greatest aspiration you can have. Living out holy sexuality isn't about holding out until you reach the "finish line" of marriage. It's about *yielding* this very personal and powerful area of your life completely and totally to the lordship of Christ. It's about *admitting* your failures and struggles to the redemptive power of Jesus. And it's about daily *depending* upon the Holy Spirit to fight the battles that you feel too weak to win.

There have been few areas of my life that have been more humbling and revealing than my sexuality. My thoughts, my attitudes, and my actions regarding sex unveil things about me that I don't like—selfishness, arrogance, and foolishness. In other words, if I try to live with sexual integrity in my own strength and determination, I will fail. And that's exactly where my Savior wants me, humble and completely dependent upon His power in my weakness. My sexuality plus surrender to the lordship of Christ equals holy sexuality.

Whether we are single or married, sexuality can be a very tangible and powerful tool for refining our character.

REFLECT AND RESPOND

Check all that apply to you personally:

__ *God is using your sexual struggles to make you humble and dependent upon His strength.*

__ *Sexuality represents a test of whether you trust God's Word or if you will give in to the cultural pressure to compromise.*

__ *God is helping you understand His grace and mercy through His forgiveness and redemption in your sexual past.*

What about You?

God's greatest good isn't for you to get married and "live happily ever after." He has much greater plans to prepare your heart and soul for eternity and to make you more like Christ—to prepare your heart and soul for eternity.

Have you ever thought about the fact that God wants to be the Lord of all of you, even your sexuality? Oftentimes we accept Him as our Savior, but hesitate when He also asks to be our Lord. We compartmentalize the areas of life He is allowed to speak into. The Lord wants His truth to profoundly change how you view your sexuality, what opinions you hold, and what choices you make. There is no such thing as a "compartmentalized" follower of Christ. Being a follower of Jesus means that we are called to yield *every* part of who we are to God's truth. We are told to love God with *all* our heart, *all* our mind, *all* our soul, and *all* our strength. We lay down our own opinions and surrender our desires in order to pursue His will and righteousness.

As you process what you've read this week, let me ask you the three personal questions I posed at the beginning of this week about sexuality and your character?

REFLECT AND RESPOND

- *Who is the boss? Do you worship God or have you mixed in the worship of self?*

- *Can you trust God with your sexuality? Do you believe His intentions for you are good?*

- *What do you most want out of your life, happiness or holiness?*

I have asked the Lord a million times why I struggled with sexual sin. I hadn't been abused as a child, I have a wonderful dad, etc. And the Lord sweetly answered one day and said, "You're a sinner saved by grace and you need to learn to lean on me. Quit trying to defeat sin on your own." It was such a relief that there isn't something wrong with me for struggling with sexual sin. I am a sinner saved by grace and in need of Jesus every day. I feel like I have often struggled with knowing God but not fully having a heart knowledge of Him. I grew up in a godly family, church, and Christian school. It always seems like I have the right answers; I find myself stopping and asking if I really do believe some of things I say. Do I have a knowledge of God like in Romans 1 but deny Him in sexuality because I want to do things my way? Worshiping Jesus in my sexuality would mean giving up funny movies that are inappropriate. It would mean saying no to lustful thoughts, even when I feel tired or alone. —Vanessa

Your past choices may reveal very different answers to these questions than what you professed. Don't worry about the past. Today is a new day . . . a day to declare with your mouth and with your actions that you want Christ to be the Lord of your life and to become more like Him.

REFLECT AND RESPOND

- *How does this week's study change your perspective of sexual struggles and temptations?*

- *How can God cause sexual struggles and temptations to work out for your good?*

- *Use what you just wrote and write a prayer to God, declaring your recommitment to His lordship in your life and particularly, your sexuality.*

PULLING IT ALL TOGETHER

Below are key truths you have read about this week, some are possible answers to the questions posed at the start of the week. Now is the time to ask yourself, "How much have I embraced this truth in my life?" After each statement, circle the number (1–5) that represents the power of this truth in your life.

- Sexuality is a realistic, tangible testing ground that unveils your heart and refines your character.

1   2   3   4   5

- The wall between your sexuality and spirituality is imaginary. Your sexual choices are spiritual choices.

1   2   3   4   5

- The moral decline of the Roman culture during Paul's time was due to the fact that they dethroned God as the Creator not due to immoral sexual choices.

1   2   3   4   5

- If you look "inward" for truth, you worship self. If you look "outward" for truth, you worship other people or rationalism. If you look "upward" for truth, you worship God. The source you rely upon reveals your god.

1   2   3   4   5

- When we reject God as the ONLY one with the authority to determine morality, we begin to compromise and make moral choices based on what "feels right."

1   2   3   4   5

- It takes faith and courage to hold to a standard of truth the world hates, but that is worship.

1   2   3   4   5

- Sexuality has put God's goodness on trial because it can appear as if His Word keeps people from happiness and fulfillment.

1   2   3   4   5

- In His wisdom and goodness, God longs for you to discover a deeper happiness that comes from fellowship with Him, a transformed life, and a grateful heart.

1   2   3   4   5

- It takes faith to trust the goodness of God when His commands cause you discomfort. Only by faith will you believe that the goodness of God calls you to rewards greater than the temporary pleasure of getting what you want right now.

1   2   3   4   5

• God's purpose for your life is that you would become a spiritual daughter, becoming like Jesus in your heart and character. Your sexuality could be one of the ways God achieves this goal in your life.

1   2   3   4   5

• Living out holy sexuality is about yielding this area completely to Christ, admitting your failures and daily depending on the Holy Spirit to fight the battles you feel too weak to win.

1   2   3   4   5

• Behind your sexuality is a greater spiritual battle prompting you to ask three important questions: (1) Who do I worship? (2) Is God really good? (3) What is God's purpose for my life?

1   2   3   4   5

Which truth did you rate the lowest? Write that truth on a 3x5 card (or on your phone) and look at it this week. Ask God to plant this truth in your heart.

Sexual

Have you ever asked yourself . . .

- *How do I determine which sexual choices are right and which are wrong?*
- *How do I navigate sexual practices that are not specifically addressed in the Bible?*
- *When facing a biblical standard that is not politically correct, how have I responded?*

This week's study, "Sexual Boundaries," will bring you clarity on these questions and more. So let's begin!

Boundaries

Do You Have Questions?

You may have decided that you want to be a woman of sexual integrity. You want your choices to be an expression of your love for God. The tricky part is how to live out that commitment. While God is clear about some of our sexual choices, there seem to be a lot of grey areas. Whenever I speak at conferences, I incorporate a live Q&A time for women to anonymously text in their questions. The most common questions from both single and married women usually relate to whether certain things are right or wrong for Christians to engage in. In other words, how do I practically live out sexual integrity? Here are a few examples of the questions I hear most often:

- *Is masturbation wrong?*
- *What does God think about homosexuality?*
- *Am I still a virgin if I've had oral sex?*
- *Is it wrong to read erotic novels like* Fifty Shades of Grey?
- *How far is too far to go in a dating relationship?*

You've probably wrestled personally with some of these questions, and there are plenty of opinions available. Ask five people you know, and you will probably hear five different answers. And let's be honest . . . we usually embrace the answer that most represents what we wanted to hear.

If you truly want your sexuality to be an expression of your love for Christ, the only opinion that matters is His. Don't even consider *my opinion*! You need to be hungry for God's truth. We learn about God's truth on sexuality and every other area of life by studying the Bible, asking for wisdom, and responding to the leading of the Holy Spirit. Sexual morality isn't about a set of rules, but about honoring the holiness of God.

REFLECT AND RESPOND

- *Read Hebrews 5:12-14. What does this passage say about how you can learn to determine right from wrong?*

- *Read James 1:5. What does this verse say about how you can become wise?*

- *Read John 16:13. What did Jesus say the Holy Spirit would do in your life?*

- *How are you currently seeking truth through the Bible, prayer, and the Holy Spirit?*

Living with sexual integrity means addressing very practical questions in everyday life. To help you apply God's wisdom, you can ask yourself three important questions to find God's opinion (also known as truth!) on any question you might have.

Question #1 — Does the Bible say it's wrong?
Question #2 — Is it consistent with God's design for sexuality?
Question #3 — Is it beneficial?

REFLECT AND RESPOND

- *What are a few grey area issues you wonder about related to sexuality?*

- *Spend some time asking the Lord to give you wisdom this week as you bring these questions before Him.*

The Bible and Sexual Boundaries

Today we will tackle the first question . . .

1. DOES THE BIBLE SAY IT'S WRONG?

I am a stranger on earth; do not hide your commands from me. My soul is consumed with longing for your laws at all times. (Ps. 119:19–20)

If you are a child of God, you are a stranger on this earth. You will not make decisions like the world does. The author of Psalm 119 understood this and he was desperate for God's instruction. God's Word became his delight because it gave him the practical answers for how to live life as a child of God on Planet Earth. God's Word can do the same for you today. It is meant to be a "lamp for [your] feet" and "a light on [your] path" (Ps. 119:105).

While the Bible doesn't specifically address every sexual question you may have, it does clearly state that some sexual activity is not acceptable to God. Let me warn you, God's Word is not "politically correct." His standard for holiness doesn't change as our cultural lens changes. This can be both comforting and disturbing at the same time.

Below is a list of the sexual practices that the Bible says are wrong, some from the Old Testament and some the New Testament. People may question whether Old Testament references still apply for Christians today since it expressed the Jewish law. After all, we no longer follow rules about not eating shellfish or being ceremonially unclean during your period. A biblical scholar could give you a sophisticated answer, but here's a simple way of thinking about it. Biblical teaching about morality in the Old Testament was repeated and reinforced by Jesus and others in the New Testament while teachings about being "clean or unclean" were not. The death of Jesus on the cross made the sacrificial system obsolete; those who trust in Christ are "clean." Even though we don't follow laws about being "ceremonial clean," our actions can still be immoral and offensive to God.

Here is a list are things that the Bible says are wrong for us to engage in:

- **Fornication**—This is a broad term for immoral sex and includes sex before marriage and sex outside of marriage. In modern language, we might call it "sleeping around" or "hooking up" (Heb. 13:4; 1 Cor. 6:18–20).

- **Adultery**—This refers to having sex with someone other than your spouse. It means breaking your wedding vows. "Do not commit adultery" is one of the Ten Commandments; Jesus broadened the definition by including "adultery of the heart" meaning that we should be faithful to our marriage vows even in our thinking (Ex. 20:14; Prov. 6:32; Matt. 5:27–28).

- **Homosexuality**—Both the Old Testament and New Testament describe homosexual activity as a perversion of God's design. It is not a sin to have homosexual temptations —we can't control what we are tempted by, but acting on that temptation is wrong in God's eyes (Lev. 18:22; 20:13; Rom. 1:18, 26–27; 1 Cor. 6:9–11).

- **Prostitution**—The world's oldest profession has never been okay with God (Lev. 19:29; Jer. 13:27; Hos. 4:10–14).

- **Lustful Passions**—This does not refer to the God-given sexual desire a married man or woman has for their spouse. It refers to unrestrained sexual desire for someone you are not married to (1 Thess. 4:3–7; Titus 3:3).

- **Obscenity and Coarse Joking**—God cares about more than what we do sexually. He wants our words to be respectful of the holy gift of sexuality (Eph. 5:4).

I'm sure you've noticed that some of these biblical standards are not politically correct. God's Word doesn't change with popular opinion, so it's important to know what the Bible actually says rather than relying on cultural interpretations. You may have some questions about some of the things on this list. If so, I encourage you to go back and study these verses more closely for yourself.

Instead of seeing God's boundaries as created to protect us, many of us see them as a means to keep us from experiencing life. God's love for us is so much bigger than we can ever imagine, and He truly wants good for our lives. His love is a Father's love—pure, unconditional, and protective. He puts boundaries in place to protect and keep us from pain, not to be a fun-hater or to make our lives difficult. In reality, following God's truth brings freedom from the pain sexual sin brings.

REFLECT AND RESPOND

- *Does anything from this list surprise you? If so, which one(s)? Explain.*

- *Why do you think God says "no" to these sexual activities?*

- *What arguments have you heard to support the sexual activities from this list?*

- *How do you respond as a Christian when God's Word is different than the world's perspective?*

I have a favorite sitcom. Doesn't everyone? A few weeks ago I was laughing along to the regular banter between the characters I know so well, when I realized what I was actually laughing at. I have watched this show for years, and it didn't hit me until that day how crude the jokes are and how their view of sexuality and intimacy is so distorted. Sleeping with friends isn't only encouraged, but seen as casual as sharing a coffee. I tried to continue to watch the show, convincing myself that maybe if I didn't laugh along it was okay. This is what God means when He tells me not to engage in obscenity or coarse joking. I continued to feel convicted. I finally surrendered the show to God and I haven't watched that sitcom since . . . and, well, I'd like to report I'm doing just fine. —Emmy

WEEK 4 · DAY 3

Designer Sex

2. IS IT CONSISTENT WITH GOD'S DESIGN FOR SEXUALITY?

Have you ever wondered about God's will for your life? Whether or not He has marriage in your future, or what job He wants you to take? There are very few verses that specifically tell you God's will for you. However, this is one of them: "It is God's will that you should be sanctified: that you should avoid sexual immorality" (1 Thess. 4:3).

In week 2, you learned about the importance of embracing God's design for sexuality. God's design is for you to live with sexual integrity. (Remember, sexual integrity is when your sexual choices accurately reflect your devotion to God and reveal the level of commitment you've made to a man.) Sexual immorality is anything that twists and abuses God's design for sexuality.

As we discussed earlier, the most common way of distorting God's design for sex is when our sexual actions are completely separate from the promise we've made to God and to a man. In other words, we express our sexuality apart from its larger relational and spiritual context. God wants you to walk with sexual integrity. The question to ask yourself then is, Does this particular "grey area" in my life represent sexual integrity?

Let's use the example of erotic literature, which took the world by storm with the *Fifty Shades of Grey* phenomenon back in 2011. While you might agree with me that pornography is a distortion of God's design for sex, your thoughts on erotic books might be different. After all, there's a story line, the fictional characters are "in love" and might even end up getting married. Erotica is written to arouse you sexually. Your sexual arousal is completely unrelated to your relational reality. As much as you may be drawn to the story line, you are not "in love" with and haven't committed your life to the fictional character you are reading about. Pornography, whether written or visual, arouses you physically apart from any relationship with the people on the screen or in the story.

Dannah Gresh and I coauthored a book called *Pulling Back the Shades* to address erotica and a woman's God-given desire for intimacy. We have heard from hundreds of women who were deceived into using porn and erotica without realizing the spiritual impact of expressing their sexuality outside of God's design.

> I've been reading *Pulling Back the Shades*, and have loved it! I want to share what I've experienced since taking to heart even just half the book and giving to God what I've struggled with for years. I don't sleep around, I even fought long and hard to wait until marriage (that has yet to happen), but always thought erotica would be okay since I'm not "doing anything." And chatting, what could be wrong with that? But you are so right . . . it escalates. Not only to porn, but to subjects that make me sick inside just to get the same "rush" as the first. It's so incredibly identical to a drug addiction, and when I read in *Pulling Back the Shades* that it's a spiritual thing, I cut myself off completely to return to the godly woman I once was. —Claire

Remember, God's design is that your sexual choices accurately reflect your commitment to Him and honor the level of commitment you have made (or haven't made) to the man in your life. You make sexual choices *not* based on how you are feeling in the moment, but by who you've chosen to become.

REFLECT AND RESPOND

- *What are some examples of how God's design has been "acceptably" distorted among Christians?*

- *Do the current choices you are making line up with who you want to become?*

- *Below, write out how you would describe to someone "God's design for sexuality."*

Sex and the Grey Areas

3. IS IT BENEFICIAL?

Not every sexual action or thought is listed in the Bible with a *yes* or *no* beside it. Some things just appear to be grey areas. For example, we know from Scripture that the full expression of sexuality is to be reserved for marriage, but what about everything leading up to it? Is it okay with God for a couple to kiss, touch each other, and fantasize about what they might do if they were married?

In his letter to the Corinthian church, Paul gave us some great standards to help us discern what to do when the Bible isn't clear: "'I have the right to do anything,' you say—but not everything is beneficial. 'I have the right to do anything'—but not everything is constructive. No one should seek their own good, but the good of others" (1 Cor. 10:23–24).

Paul is saying that some things we have the freedom to do are not good for us and can also be a stumbling block to the people we love. For example, I am free to go to a movie theater and see whatever movie I want. But some movies I choose to watch are going to hurt my mind and my relationship with God. Other movies may be okay for me, but they would cause someone I love to stumble. As the mom of three teenage boys and the founder of a ministry that talks about sexual issues, I have to be very careful that my choices don't hurt other people.

You might not be in ministry, but your choices impact people around you. While you may not be breaking the rules with your boyfriend, some things you choose to do together may be harmful for one or both of you. Passionate kissing might not tempt you, but if it tempts your boyfriend to go further sexually, these actions are not "beneficial" to him or to your relationship. I'm guessing you've probably done things with a guy in the past and regret giving so much of yourself to him, even if you didn't have intercourse. Even if something isn't specifically listed in the Bible as a sin, it can still be harmful, selfish, and unloving.

God is not about us simply following a list of rules. He wants us to seek His wisdom and honor Him in every choice we make. His desire is for you to make wise choices to keep yourself and others from emotional and spiritual harm.

> Our physical relationship was progressing faster than I expected. But when I couldn't find specific examples in Scripture saying no to things like oral sex, I assumed it was okay as long as we weren't having intercourse. Each time I was intimate with my boyfriend, I would leave the situation feeling shameful and dirty. Why did I feel this way if it wasn't wrong? This shame pushed me away from God, and I found myself avoiding prayer and devotion time. I knew what God wanted me to do, but I didn't want to hear it. I realize now how much this hurt my relationship with my boyfriend and with God. I should have invited God into this discussion instead of shutting Him out. —Carmen

REFLECT AND RESPOND

- *Why do you think God leaves some sexual choices to your discretion rather than clearly saying "no"?*

- *Is it difficult for you to ask God for wisdom about sexual decisions? If so why?*

Getting Practical

Today, let's take a few common "grey areas" and run them through the "three question grid." Probably the question single women most often ask about is whether or not masturbation is wrong.

Take a few moments as a group to discuss these three questions as they relate to the issue of masturbation (without sharing personal stories or examples). If you are doing this study alone, perhaps take some time to think it over quietly.

1. Does the Bible say masturbation is wrong?

Nowhere in Scripture is the concept of masturbation even mentioned. For certain, it was an issue for men and women in biblical times, so why doesn't God include teaching that says, "Thou shalt not . . ."?

While the Bible doesn't address the issue specifically, it does tell us not to entertain lustful thoughts (1 Thess. 4:3–5; Matt. 5:28). Masturbation is typically, but not always, linked to sexual fantasies and/or pornography. What are the implications of this?

2. Is masturbation consistent with God's design for sexuality?

Sexuality was intended to be fully expressed between a man and a woman in the covenant of marriage. Is self-pleasuring consistent with that design?

Some Christian teachers encourage singles to use masturbation as a means of curbing sexual temptation so that sex can be saved for marriage. Others point out that sex was never intended to be for "self-pleasure" but to bring pleasure to your spouse. What do you think?

3. Is masturbation helpful to your walk with God?

I've met many men and women who learned to rely on masturbation to cope with stress, depression, loneliness, and boredom. Paired with fantasy or pornography, masturbation can become addictive. Unfortunately, some men and women have sexual difficulties in marriage because they have become so reliant on self-pleasure.

Although masturbation isn't specifically labeled as "sinful," it presents some traps that can foster temptation rather than keeping you from it. Many women are burdened by tremendous guilt and shame because of a struggle with masturbation. God knows that you are a sexual woman with a body that is mature and longing for intimacy. There is nothing sinful about your longings for sexual intimacy, nor is there anything shameful about your physical desires. Jesus probably faced similar temptations as we're told in Hebrews 4:15: "For we do not have a high priest who is unable to sympathize with our weaknesses, but one who in every respect has been tempted as we are, yet without sin" (ESV). The struggle isn't the issue, it's what you do about it that matters. Do you take your struggle to God for His wisdom or do you hide it from Him?

Masturbation is a personal and complicated issue that each woman has to ask the Lord about. When God wanted to be clear about something, He inspired clear teaching in Scripture. The Bible is silent on masturbation. What God *did* state definitely is that He wants to give us His wisdom. "If any of you lacks wisdom, you should ask God, who gives generously to all without finding fault, and it will be given to you" (James 1:5).

Below is another example for you to work through. A young woman recently asked me this question:

> *Does God really leave sexual choices to our discretion? I never would have thought that. I'm struggling a lot with what's acceptable and what's not. My boyfriend and I are struggling to figure this out. We want our relationship to be founded on God, but what sexual choices are okay? For example, oral sex. I don't know what God thinks about it and I would never even consider talking to my mom! How do we know where to draw the line? —Janell*

What advice would you give this young woman? Run her question through the "three questions grid" from this chapter.

1. Does the Bible say oral sex (outside of marriage) is wrong? Has God said no?

God has said that fornication (sex outside of marriage) is wrong. Is oral sex considered a sexual act in God's eyes?

2. Is having oral sex with your boyfriend consistent with God's design?

God's design is for you to live with sexual integrity. (Remember, sexual integrity is when your sexual choices accurately reflect your devotion to God and reveal the level of commitment you've made to a man.) Are you able to live with sexual integrity while also having oral sex with your boyfriend? Is this sexual act a "consistent reflection of your relational and spiritual commitments"?

3. Is this act beneficial to you, to your boyfriend, and to your community?

Does it help you in your walk with the Lord? Is it a good testimony or is it a stumbling block?

A big piece of yielding your sexuality to the Lord is asking for His wisdom in these very personal questions. When God has been clear in His Word, obey Him even if you don't understand His reasoning. When God hasn't been clear, ask Him to guide you!

The purpose of this week's lesson wasn't to make you feel guilty for past mistakes but to help you make better choices moving forward. The world definitely has its own "wisdom" about sexuality, but "the wisdom of this world is foolishness to God" (1 Cor. 3:19 NLT).

Regardless of how you've made choices in the past, you can choose today to embrace God's wisdom. Your enemy will always try to convince you that your past defines you. Have you heard his deceptive whispers? *You already had sex, it's too late to be pure in God's eyes. . . . God can't forgive what you have done. . . . You have already gone this far, one step further won't hurt.* See these whispers for what they are—lies—and instead let God's truth about you sink in. You are forgiven. It's time to move forward.

REFLECT AND RESPOND

- *How does God's wisdom on sexuality conflict with what you've learned from worldly wisdom?*

- *What are some things in your life that God is calling you to give up or abandon to seek righteousness and purity in Him?*

- *Take what you just wrote and write a prayer to God. Lay this area of your life before Him and express your commitment from this day forward.*

PULLING IT ALL TOGETHER

Below are key truths you have read about this week that also answer the questions posed at the start of the week. Now is the time to ask yourself, "How much have I embraced this truth in my life?" After each statement, circle the number (1–5) that represents the power of this truth in your life.

- If I truly want my sexuality to be an expression of my love for Christ, the only opinion that matters is His.

1   2   3   4   5

- If I am a child of God I will not make decisions like the world does. When looking for God's truth on sexual choices, I need to ask myself three important questions. Does the Bible say it's wrong? Is it consistent with God's design for sexuality? Is it beneficial?

1   2   3   4   5

- Some biblical standards are not politically correct. God's Word doesn't change with popular opinion, so know what the Bible is saying rather than relying on cultural interpretations.

1   2   3   4   5

- First Corinthians 10:23-24 says that some things I have the freedom to do are not good for me and can also be a stumbling block to the people I love.

1   2   3   4   5

- Even if something isn't specifically listed in the Bible as a sin, it can still be harmful, selfish, and unloving.

1   2   3   4   5

- When God has been clear in His Word, I need to obey Him even if I don't understand His reasoning. When God hasn't been clear, I must ask Him to guide me!

1   2   3   4   5

- Regardless of how I've made choices in the past, I can choose today to embrace God's wisdom. The enemy will always try to convince me that my past defines me. I am forgiven. It's time to move forward.

1   2   3   4   5

Which truth did you rate the lowest? Write that truth on a 3x5 card (or on your phone) and look at it this week. Ask God to plant this truth in your heart.

Battling

Have you ever asked yourself . . .

- *Where does temptation stem from?*
- *Once I feel tempted, what should I do?*
- *Are there practical steps I can take to resist temptation?*
- *Do I currently have an effective strategy to fight temptation?*

This week's study, "Battling Temptation," will bring you clarity on these questions and more. So, here we go!

Temptation

Understanding Temptation

A woman recently sent me this email:

> *Cursed be the day I was created . . .*
> *I hate the fact that I am still struggling with porn . . .*
> *I hate it with a passion . . .*
> *No longer do tears run down my cheeks because of repentance, but rather hate . . .*
> *Juli, I hate this!*
> *I've prayed so much about this, I had counseling two semesters ago, I installed Covenant Eyes, I need a miracle . . . I am losing my faith over this stupid struggle that I face!*

Perhaps, like this woman, you find yourself identifying with what Paul wrote, "I don't really understand myself, for I want to do what is right, but I don't do it. Instead, I do what I hate. . . . What a miserable person I am!" (Rom. 7:15, 24 NLT). Every man and woman can relate to feeling this way. Whether it is sexual sin or some other temptation, we fight a daily battle to pursue holiness. How terrible it feels to fall into sin once we've determined to say "no"!

No one sets out to fall into temptation, but every one of us has. It's key to understand that the foundation of sexual temptation is the natural, God-given desire for something good. You were created for deep, *yada* knowing! Your desire to express your sexuality is a good thing. Satan takes that holy desire and presents you with shortcuts—counterfeits that appear to meet the longings of your heart but end up in hurt, rejection, and shame. Every one of us—single or married—is vulnerable to counterfeit intimacy. Sex before marriage, fantasies, sexual chat rooms, erotic novels, and pornography are a few of the ways that we can fall into the trap.

A PEEK AT THE ENEMY'S PLAYBOOK

Several years ago, a major league sports team was caught cheating by filming the defensive signals of their opponents. This meant that they knew their opponent's game plan before the game began. By knowing the other team's strategy, they could successfully defend against it.

What this sports team did was unethical because it gave them an unfair advantage. However, these same rules *don't* apply to us as we stand against our adversary. We are not playing a game; we are in a war.

Have you ever considered that your heart—even your sexuality—represents a battle-field? As much as God wants to redeem this area of your life, Satan wants to destroy you through it. The name "Satan" literally means "adversary." He is God's adversary and he is yours. How many countless lives has he ruined through twisting sexuality?

In His grace, God has given us a peek at the enemy's playbook. The Bible contains many stories and passages that tell us how our adversary will try to entice us to sin. In the passage below, we see four steps of how we move from temptation into sin and destruction.

And remember, when you are being tempted, do not say, "God is tempting me." God is never tempted to do wrong, and he never tempts anyone else. Temptation comes from our own desires, which entice us and drag us away. These desires give birth to sinful actions. And when sin is allowed to grow, it gives birth to death. (James 1:13–15 NLT)

Here are the four stages:

> Stage 1: We feel a desire.
> Stage 2: We linger in the desire.
> Stage 3: We take the bait.
> Stage 4: We experience death.

Have you ever found yourself in sin and wondered, "How did I get here? I never wanted to end up here!" James's teaching helps us understand how we go from being tempted to the place of despair after jumping into sin.

REFLECT AND RESPOND

- *Reread James 1:13-15. Where does your temptation come from?*

- *Now go back and reread those verses a third time, circling the four stages that lead you into sin.*

- *Which one of the four stages do you think is your best bet in winning the battle against temptation? Why?*

The Progression of Temptation

As we read yesterday, James 1:13–15 helped us understand how we go from being tempted to the place of despair after jumping into sin. The four stages into sin again are:

> Stage 1: We feel a desire.
> Stage 2: We linger in the desire.
> Stage 3: We take the bait.
> Stage 4: We experience death.

James says that *temptation* begins with our own desires (Stage 1). While your desire may come out of a healthy place, temptation tells you that you can compromise or take a "shortcut" to get what you desire. For example, you may be craving the experience of sexual intimacy within a dating relationship. Temptation tells you, "God hasn't brought marriage. How long are you going to wait? You don't have to wait to have sex."

Let's play out a scenario to show you what I mean . . .

Alex is 28 and is attending her college roommate's wedding. Of all her college friends, she is the only one who is still single. As hard as she tries to be happy at the wedding, her heart is heavy with the burden of her singleness. She wants more than anything to be a wife, and it has been excruciating to watch this come true for everyone in her life except her. Alex is currently seeing someone, but knows deep down he isn't who she wants to marry. She has settled for his company in her loneliness and convinces herself it is only temporary. At the wedding reception, twisting her fork in her cake, Alex's mind wanders . . . she becomes jealous for what her friend and her new husband get to experience that night. She would give anything to feel that intimacy with someone.

The second stage of temptation is lingering in desires. My mentor, Linda Dillow, once told me, "You can't control what comes into your mind, but you can control what stays there." James says we are "dragged away" with the thought of having what we want. We convince ourselves that we deserve what we want or that it's not a big deal to compromise sexually. Or we reason, "I've already lost my sexual purity so what does it matter if I do it one more time."

As her thoughts consume her, Alex begins to think that since God hasn't brought her marriage, she shouldn't have to wait for intimacy. She looks over at her wedding date and begins to fantasize. She could have what her friend is having. She has the man, and she knows he would be willing to go further sexually. "What would it hurt to test the waters? We don't have to have sex . . . but maybe we could take our physical relationship to the next level . . ."

As we linger, we eventually choose to *take the bait* and to step into sin, which is Stage 3. There is a very fine and definite line between being tempted and choosing to sin. If you think back to your own sin struggles, you can probably identify when you took this step into sin.

Alex feels excited and in control. She has been waiting so long to feel intimate with someone, and the thought that it could happen that night is exhilarating. Although her emotions and hormones are flying high, Alex also knows better. She looks to her left to see her date. With a simple touch or word, she could step into her fantasy. She looks to her right and sees her good friend. She knows if she shares with her friend what she is feeling, her friend will remind her of God's truth and encourage her not to make a foolish decision based on temporary pleasure. Alex is at a crossroads. She can choose to act on her temptation or to flee.

Finally, temptation leads to *death* (Stage 4). The crossroads of temptation is not just a choice between sin and righteousness, but between life and death. Death doesn't always mean that we experience a physical death. James is also referring to the loss of intimacy with God, the loss of your dignity or the death of your testimony. We all know that sick feeling of remorse and regret when we've stepped into sin. As much as we might try to push away those feelings, sin leads to spiritual death. You might think that is overstating it, but God's Word spells out this truth.

REFLECT AND RESPOND

- *List out/rewrite the four stages of temptation.*

- *What could Alex have done to stop the temptation at Stage 1 or 2 instead of letting it progress?*

- *How did Alex linger in the desire? Go back into the scenario and underline the words or phrases that reveal she was lingering.*

- *How have you seen this progression play out in your own life?*

Preparing for Temptation

Did you know that you can prepare today for temptation that may come tomorrow? Peter wrote, "Be alert and of sober mind. Your enemy the devil prowls around like a roaring lion looking for someone to devour" (1 Peter 5:8). That's a scary thought! What if we could see the spiritual reality of the devil prowling around us, ready to pounce? If I could see this spiritual reality, I would probably be more intentional about bracing myself for temptation and testing.

What do you think Peter means by being "alert and of sober mind"? I think it means we can be proactive in preparing for temptation before it even hits us. The night before Jesus was arrested and crucified He warned His disciples, and Peter specifically, about coming temptation. His advice was, "Watch and pray so that you will not fall into temptation. The spirit is willing, but the flesh is weak" (Matt. 26:41). These are Jesus' words urging us not to just watch for a day or pray every now and then but keep on watching and praying. Why? Because temptation is sure to come again when we least expect it. We need to develop a lifestyle, expecting that our enemy is on the prowl like a roaring lion, looking for someone to devour. Today we will look at three specific strategies we can implement to be on our guard for coming temptation.

STRATEGY #1: STOP FLIRTING WITH SIN.

Imagine that you are at the zoo watching the lions who are on the other side of a trench filled with water. The lions are beautiful and majestic. Basking in the sunlight, they look tame and even peaceful. You are mesmerized by their beauty and tranquility and you want to get a better look. You climb on top of the barrier that separates you from the lions. You carefully climb to the edge of the trench, thinking the lions couldn't possibly traverse the water. You, my friend, are flirting with death. As peaceful as they may look, those lions are deadly.

This is how we often flirt with sin. It seems harmless to inch up to the edge of the trench. You won't look at hard-core porn, but you will linger on a sexually charged dating site. You won't get naked with a guy, but you let him put his hands all over you. Just like that lion could pounce at any time, so could overwhelming temptation when we take it lightly.

King Josiah lived in a time when Israel was entrenched in pagan worship. Josiah brought reform and revival because he took sin (and all of its trappings) very seriously.

REFLECT AND RESPOND

• *Read the account of Josiah's reform in 2 Chronicles 34:*

In the eighth year of his reign, while he was still young, he began to seek the God of his father David. In his twelfth year he began to purge Judah and Jerusalem of high places, Asherah poles and idols. Under his direction the altars of the Baals were torn down; he cut to pieces the incense altars that were above them, and smashed the Asherah poles and the idols. These he broke to pieces and scattered over the graves of those who had sacrificed to them. He burned the bones of the priests on their altars, and so he purged Judah and Jerusalem. In the towns of Manasseh, Ephraim and Simeon, as far as Naphtali, and in the ruins around them, he tore down the altars and the Asherah poles and crushed the idols to powder and cut to pieces all the incense altars throughout Israel." (2 Chron. 34:3-7)

• *Underline all of the action verbs in the passage above that show how Josiah destroyed the idols that were causing the Israelites to sin.*

• *How do you "flirt with sin"?*

• *What would a radical pursuit of purity (like Josiah's actions) look like in your life?*

STRATEGY #2: PUT ON THE ARMOR OF GOD.

Below is the most famous passage on how to prepare for a spiritual battle. Paul wrote this encouragement to the young Christians in the church in Ephesus, but its message is for us today as we face temptation. In this passage, Paul lists several metaphorical but true spiritual weapons we can use to stand against our enemy.

> Finally, be strong in the Lord and in his mighty power. Put on the full armor of God, so that you can take your stand against the devil's schemes. For our struggle is not against flesh and blood, but against the rulers, against the authorities, against the powers of this dark world and against the spiritual forces of evil in the heavenly realms. Therefore put on the full armor of God, so that when the day of evil comes, you may be able to stand your ground, and after you have done everything, to stand. Stand firm then, with the belt of truth buckled around your waist, with the breastplate of righteousness in place, and with your feet fitted with the readiness that comes from the gospel of peace. In addition to all this, take up the shield of faith, with which you can extinguish all the flaming arrows of the evil one. Take the helmet of salvation and the sword of the Spirit, which is the word of God.
>
> And pray in the Spirit on all occasions with all kinds of prayers and requests. With this in mind, be alert and always keep on praying for all the Lord's people. (Eph. 6:10–18)

REFLECT AND RESPOND

How can you "put on" this armor in real life?

• *The belt of truth:* _____

• *The breastplate of righteousness:* _____

- *The readiness of the gospel of peace:* _____

- *The shield of faith:* _____

- *The helmet of salvation:* _____

- *The sword of the Spirit:* _____

- *Constantly praying in the Spirit:* _____

STRATEGY #3: DON'T BE SPIRITUALLY ISOLATED.

Read this wisdom from Ecclesiastes 4:

> Two are better than one, because they have a good return for their labor:
> If either of them falls down, one can help the other up.
> But pity anyone who falls and has no one to help them up.
> Also, if two lie down together, they will keep warm. But how can one keep warm alone?
> Though one may be overpowered, two can defend themselves.
> A cord of three strands is not quickly broken. (Ecc. 4:9–12)

REFLECT AND RESPOND

- *What does this passage say about the importance of fighting temptation with help rather than alone?*

- *Who in your life helps you battle temptation? If no one, who could you ask?*

- *How can you be more proactive in sharing your temptation with people who can help you and encourage you?*

• *Take a few minutes and review the three strategies for being "on your guard." Which one do you need to spend more time focusing on?*

When I decided to take a stand against my addiction to porn and masturbation, I knew I would have to change my lifestyle to keep myself from slipping up. I determined it wasn't healthy for me to be alone in my dorm room, especially at night or if I was stressed out. I created a plan and steps I would take to avoid these situations—walks with friends, inviting friends over, doing my homework in common areas, and avoiding watching shows and movies with sexual content. I also found new, healthier ways to relieve stress, like working out and spending time in prayer and solitude. **—Kelsey**

Responding to Temptation

Not only has God given us a glimpse into Satan's strategies, He has also given specific instruction on how to stand against temptation when it hits us square on the nose. Yesterday we looked at Peter's reminder for us to be on guard and sober minded because Satan is like a prowling lion, seeking someone to devour. In the next verse, Peter tells us what to do when we actually encounter the lion. "Resist him, standing firm in the faith, because you know that the family of believers throughout the world is undergoing the same kind of sufferings" (1 Peter 5:9).

Other passages in the Bible help us to develop specific strategies of what exactly to do when temptation comes. One of my favorites is 1 Corinthians 10:13: "No temptation has overtaken you except what is common to mankind. And God is faithful; he will not let you be tempted beyond what you can bear. But when you are tempted, he will also provide a way out so that you can endure it."

REFLECT AND RESPOND

- *What does this passage tell you about sin and temptation?*

- *What specific advice does Paul give about how you should respond to temptation?*

• *This passage gives four truths (or promises) to use as you combat the lies Satan feeds you about your struggle with temptation. List out the four promises you read in 1 Corinthians 10:13.*

Here are some very practical steps you can implement when temptation comes your way.

Step #1: Remember that you are not alone.

Both Paul and Peter mention that other Christians around the world are going through similar temptations and trials as you experience.

Most likely you are learning through this study that other friends in your community have some of the same temptations that you face. Satan would love for you to believe that you are the only Christian who has your past or faces your specific temptations. Reminding yourself that your temptations are not unique can give you courage to reach out to a friend for help. There are many other women around the world who know exactly how you feel and who are engaged in the same battle you are currently fighting.

Step #2: Don't let the temptation define you.

It is interesting to me how many characters in the Gospels (the books that record Jesus' life on earth) are defined by their sin and not even given a name. We meet tax collectors, prostitutes, and sorcerers . . . each defined by his or her sin when they first encounter Jesus. Jesus often gives them a new identity (and sometimes a new name). One of the ways Satan can discourage you is to link your identity with your temptation or your past sin.

In 1 Corinthians 6, Paul lists the kind of people who will not enter the kingdom of God including the sexually immoral, thieves, prostitutes, and greedy people. Then Paul writes, "And that is what some of you *were*. But you were washed, you were sanctified, you were justified in the name of the Lord Jesus Christ and by the Spirit of our God" (1 Cor. 6:11, emphasis mine).

If you are a child of God, your temptations and/or past sins should never define you.

When you allow your temptations to become a part of your identity, they hold more power over you. If you are a child of God, that alone is your identity regardless of the labels the world may give you. In today's culture, it is common to identify yourself by sexual orientation or gender preferences. We often hear things like, "I identify as LGBTQ." While this may be culturally encouraged, a Christian's identity can not be primarily based on sexuality or sexual orientation. If you are same-sex attracted, that may be a struggle or a temptation, but it is *not* your identity in Christ. Remember . . . you are washed, sanctified, and justified.

Step #3: Find the way of escape.

God promises that He will provide a way of escaping every temptation, but are you looking for it? Maybe your "way of escape" is to call a friend or to firmly declare, "I'm NOT going there! That's not who I am." You never *have* to sin! Don't fall for the lie that you don't have a choice.

Step #4: Flee!

What do you think it means to flee? It means to run as fast as you can from the temptation. It means to run away from whatever could cause you to sin. If you are in a compromising relationship, run from it! If your iPhone is your portal for porn, get an old-fashioned flip phone. Maybe you have to physically run away like Joseph did as we saw in Genesis 39.

REFLECT AND RESPOND

- *Why do you think it's important to remember you are not alone when you are tempted?*

- *How can you rely on your friends when you are tempted in the future?*

- *How have you let your temptations or past define you?*

- *List some practical examples of how God has provided you a way of escape in the past.*

Creating an Action Plan

We have covered a lot of ground this week! On days 1 and 2, we looked at how temptation progresses. On day 3, we learned how to prepare for future temptation. Yesterday, we learned what to do when you are in the midst of temptation. Today, we are going to bring all of this information together to create an action plan for addressing sexual temptation. Satan has a plan. So should you!

Action Step #1: Be honest about your vulnerability.

While temptations may pop up out of nowhere, Satan typically attacks us in our weakness. There are certain sins we find ourselves falling in again and again. We also have "triggers" that set us up for temptation. Identifying the trigger and the temptation can help you be alert and on your guard. Below, list two or three specific areas of sexual temptation and triggers you struggle with.

- I'm tempted to _____
  when _____ (trigger).

- I'm tempted to _____
  when _____ (trigger).

- I'm tempted to _____
  when _____ (trigger).

Action Step #2: Use spiritual weapons.

Your primary spiritual weapons are prayer and knowing God's Word. Jesus resisted Satan in the desert by reciting Scripture back to him. If this was Jesus' strategy and He was sinless, then we'd be wise to do the same! Below, write out a specific strategy to use these weapons in your battle with temptation.

• How will you use the weapon of prayer?

• How will you use the weapon of knowing and/or memorizing God's Word?

Action Step #3: Build your community.

Write down the name of a friend or mentor you trust to be a "flee friend." A "flee friend" is someone you can call for wisdom and help in the midst of temptation. Contact this person and ask them to be your "flee friend," someone you can count on to remind you of God's truth when temptation comes knocking. If you are dealing with a temptation, tell a friend, and tell them today!

• My "flee friend" is _____.

Write down the name of an older woman who is a mentor to you. A mentor is someone who has a deep walk with the Lord and has been through some of the battles you are facing. If you don't have a mentor, begin asking God to bring you one.

• My mentor is _____.

What helped me wait until my wedding night to be sexually active? Was it a stellar sense of self-worth? Maybe self-control made out of steel? No, neither of those. Sure, some might blame it on the fact that I am a firstborn—you know . . . the responsible, rule-following type. But it goes much deeper than that. What led me to make countercultural choices was primarily one thing, godly mentors who were Jesus-with-skin-on to me. My relationship with Christ and these godly influences proved to be my anchor as I navigated the sex-saturated culture.
—Abby

I cannot express how important it is to have a "flee friend." I would even be bold enough to say that you probably will not completely defeat and walk away from a temptation without one. I also cannot express how grateful I am for my "flee friend"! She has had to say difficult things for me to hear and I have not always been happy with her but I am beyond blessed to have an honest and trustworthy sister in Christ in my life. One of my biggest struggles is texting, talking, seeing, and hooking up with men. She is willing to ask who I am talking to and what are we talking about, why are we talking, etc. She has permission to check through my cell phone if she asks. A rule I have put into place for myself is to not answer a text or call if the number is not programmed into my phone and to delete that message on the spot. A lot of men in my past have my number and I don't need to talk to any of them! I also (in general) do not text any guys after 8 or 9 p.m. —Vanessa

Action Step #4: Identify your way of escape.

You learned this week that God always provides a way of escape when you face temptation. Sometimes the "escape hatch" just means running away like Joseph did when Potiphar's wife tried to seduce him. Other times the "escape hatch" means walking away from a friendship that encourages sin or planning positive activities (like exercise, calling a friend, or putting on worship music) when loneliness triggers sexual temptation. What are some "escape hatches" you can use when you feel tempted?

- When I am tempted by _____
  I will _____.

- When I am tempted by _____
  I will _____.

Action Step #5: Remember who guards you.

A few years ago, I was struggling with a temptation that I just couldn't seem to overcome. To make matters worse, the Lord put me in a position that was full of triggers for my temptation. I asked the Lord to remove me from the situation. Instead, He showed me a benediction (or statement of praise) closing the book of Jude that has been a great encouragement to me:

To him who is able to keep you from stumbling and to present you before his glorious presence without fault and with great joy—to the only God our Savior be glory, majesty, power and authority, through Jesus Christ our Lord, before all ages, now and forevermore! Amen. (Jude 24–25)

It's my responsibility to seek the Lord with my temptations and weaknesses, but only He is able to keep me from stumbling. I'm learning every day to trust the Lord to be strong within me as I battle sin and temptation.

- What does it mean for me to trust the Lord to keep me from stumbling?

- Write your own benediction (statement of praise) remembering who is able to keep you from falling.

My benediction:

Below is the "action plan" one woman developed as she went through the pilot study:

- **I will stop flirting with sin.** I need to be honest about how tempting it is to be alone with my boyfriend. We have already crossed some lines we shouldn't have. We need to get serious about setting boundaries. I will have this conversation with my boyfriend.

- **I will use spiritual weapons.** I need to spend time in prayer and worship asking the Lord about these things. He cares and will lead me to make decisions that will protect me.

- **I am building my community.** I will be honest with my friends about my temptations. I have asked Stacie to be my "flee friend," and I am asking God to bring me a mentor to ask me hard questions and pray with me.

- **I have identified my ways of escape.** I realize that part of my "way of escape" is in how I prepare. I don't want to be alone with my boyfriend in the evening. We can spend time at a coffee shop instead of his apartment. I will text Stacie when we get in the car so I'm not tempted to be alone there for long periods of time.

- **I will remember who guards me.** Lord, thank You that all is not lost, even if I fall or continue to struggle. Thank You that guilt and shame don't have to determine my future. I praise You that Your forgiveness is full and free and You can keep me from falling!

PULLING IT ALL TOGETHER

Below are key truths you have read about this week that also answer the questions posed at the start of the week. Now is the time to ask yourself, "How much have I embraced this truth in my life?"

After each statement, circle the number (1–5) that represents the power of this truth in your life.

- The foundation of sexual temptation is the natural, God-given desire for something good. Satan takes that holy desire and presents me with short-cuts—counterfeits that appear to meet the longings of my heart but end up in hurt, rejection, and shame.

1   2   3   4   5

- James 1:13–15 lays out four steps I move through from temptation into sin and destruction.

1   2   3   4   5

- While my desire may come out of a healthy place, temptation tells me that I can compromise or take a "shortcut" to get what I desire.

1   2   3   4   5

- While I can't control what comes into my mind, allowing a thought to linger is in my control.

1   2   3   4   5

- Lingering thoughts often lead me to choose to take the bait and step into sin.

1   2   3   4   5

- Temptation leads to death. Death doesn't always mean a physical death but could mean the loss of intimacy with God, my dignity, or my testimony.

1   2   3   4   5

- The crossroads of temptation is not just a choice between sin and righteousness, but between life and death.

1   2   3   4   5

- Temptation is common to everyone. I should expect it to come, not let it define me, look for the way of escape, and run from anything that could cause me to sin.

1   2   3   4   5

- I need to develop a lifestyle of prayer and accountability because I know the enemy is on the prowl and is looking to devour me.

1   2   3   4   5

- Both temptation and God's strength to resist it are guarantees!

1   2   3   4   5

Which truth did you rate the lowest? Write that truth on a 3x5 card (or on your phone) and look at it this week. Ask God to plant this truth in your heart.

Restoring

Have you ever asked yourself . . .

- *Why do I hide my sin from God and others?*
- *What role does the enemy play in the keeping of shameful secrets?*
- *Are sexual sins different from other sins?*
- *How do I let go of my mental list of sins?*
- *What does freedom from sin look like? Do I live that way?*
- *What does it mean to have a new identity in Christ? Do I live that way?*

This week's study, "Restoring Intimacy with God," will bring you clarity on these questions and more.

Intimacy with God

Breaking Down the Barriers

I know God forgives sins, but my sins feel too heavy. I've made promises to God over and over again only to break them. I feel weak and dirty.

I love getting the attention of guys through my body. It's like I can't say "no" when a guy shows interest in me. Every time I've gotten into a new relationship, I tell God that I will set boundaries, but things always seem to go too far. In the moment, I feel beautiful and powerful, but then I wake up in a pile of shame. I've stopped going to church and no one knows what I'm struggling with. I don't know what to do with my relationship with God. Even if He would forgive, I can't trust myself to change. I'm too ashamed to even think about God, the Bible, or church. —Madison

Like Madison, you may experience your sexuality as something that has kept you from intimacy with God. Guilt over your current or past sexual choices feels like a wall between you and God. You may be reading words about how Jesus loves you, but they just don't feel real.

Maybe through this study you've gotten a glimpse of how choosing to live with sexual integrity can actually draw you into a deeper relationship with God. Yet there are still barriers to making that a reality. Every woman has had barriers between herself and God. In fact, the main message of the entire Bible is God's plan to break down the barriers that stand between His holy love and the people He created to be His own.

Over the years, I've met hundreds of women, young and old, who don't believe they can ever experience a truly intimate relationship with God. They may read the Bible and even serve God in a variety of missions. Even so, the idea of knowing God is a foreign concept.

REFLECT AND RESPOND

- *How would you describe your personal relationship with God?*

- *What barriers do you feel stand in the way of you actually knowing God?*

- *Read 2 Corinthians 10:4-5. What are the spiritual strongholds specifically designed to keep you from? How do you tear down these strongholds?*

The greatest barrier to knowing God is our sin. It is a spiritual fact—God is holy and we are not. While we may talk about Jesus dying on the cross to erase the barrier of sin, living in the freedom of forgiveness is quite a different thing.

I've met many Christian women who understand the concept of forgiveness but still don't *feel forgiven*. This is particularly true related to sexual sin.

There is something unique about sexual sins. They seem to "stick" to us in a different way than other sins. For example, if you gossiped about a friend five years ago, you probably don't remember that today. But if you had sex with a guy five years ago, chances are you remember it. Sexual sins often wound us and other people, but that does *not* mean that sexual sins are unforgivable. Jesus died to set you free from sin, period!

REFLECT AND RESPOND

- *Read Proverbs 6:16-19. This passage lists seven sins the Lord hates. Rewrite them in your own words. Are you surprised that none of these sins are specifically sexual?*

- *Do you assume sexual sin is worse (or harder for God to cleanse) than other sins? Why?*

I recently asked a friend of mine to share a bit about her personal journey to shake the sexual sin from her past. She has been married for several years, but the guilt and shame from her past as a single woman have haunted her in her sexual relationship with her husband. Below are my questions and her candid responses:

Q: When did you first realize that your past mistakes were impacting intimacy in your marriage?

A: It's hard to pinpoint the moment when I clearly understood my past mistakes were impacting my marriage. In some way, I knew I craved a deeper level of communication and intimacy with my husband but I struggled to understand why we hadn't achieved it. During a particularly difficult season in our marriage, I began to prayerfully consider the role I played in allowing those obstacles to remain a part of our relationship. God showed me, over time, that my guilt and shame were overshadowing the beautiful relationship He desired to create in our marriage. It became clear that my choices, made long before we married, were now creating a sticky mess of emotion in the very relationship I wanted desperately to protect and honor.

Q: Can you describe the guilt you felt and how that played out in daily life?

A: My feelings of guilt and negativity were so powerful. They encompassed much of my private thought life and Satan had me nearly believing that I was one of the few Christian women who hadn't saved herself for marriage. The misconceptions seemed to take on a life of their own: if I couldn't give my husband my purity, then everything else I did—no matter how I loved him—was inadequate. In many ways, I became so fixated on that lie that I began to wonder whether I could ever be the wife my husband deserved.

Q: As a Christian, how did you accept the forgiveness of Christ while being unable to truly embrace the reality of that forgiveness?

A: For years, Satan convinced me that sexual sin is somehow different from all other sins—that choices like mine can't be redeemed. I struggled mightily to accept that

God's grace extended to my reality. After all, I hadn't been abused, I hadn't been forced to compromise my body; I chose it—and I chose it despite all of the good teaching of my parents and my faith.

This season of struggle brought me squarely back to the foot of the cross. During that time, God challenged me to find in Scripture even one example of His limiting the gift of forgiveness. I looked and looked, but never found one. Instead, I rediscovered the blessing of boundless grace. God reminded me that His mercies are new *every* morning and that reality forced me to believe that God hasn't segmented my sins. He's forgiven them all and He has called me to live a life worthy of that gift.

Q: What was it that helped you break free from the guilt?

A: The journey to move past the guilt has been long; six years into my marriage, I'm still walking the road toward freedom. I have seen my greatest progress during those times when I intentionally focus on who I am as a daughter of the Most High King. In His eyes, I am blameless, free, and forgiven; I am beautiful and worthy. His promises and His Word remind me of His truth; they also teach me that God can redeem my broken choices and transform my marriage into one that reflects His love.

Q: What one piece of advice would you give to women who are struggling with past sexual sin?

A: Own it. Own the reality of your past mistakes; own the role you played in choosing less than God's best for your life, and own the fact that those choices will be part of your life forever. Then, own grace. Own forgiveness and own the promise that God will use all things for His glory—even those sins that may feel too shameful for His mercy.

My friend shared her struggle so that you might also walk this journey of freedom in your sexuality, in your singleness or in marriage. This week's study will dig deeper into *how* we live in this freedom!

Coming Out of Hiding

Did you ever play hide and seek as a kid? I grew up in an old English tudor that had hundreds of great hiding places. Hide and seek isn't the only hiding game we first learned as children. Before we were even aware of it, we were taught subtly or overtly that some things should be kept secret. No one had to tell you to bury the shame of sexual abuse, your struggle with porn, masturbating, or cutting. You just intuitively knew that not all truth should be exposed.

All of us know, to some extent, the stress and duplicity of living a "double life." There is the confident Christian on the outside who knows the right words to speak and how to act. But there is also the secret self who has thoughts and desires that we never want to admit. Sometimes we even create two sets of friends—those who interact with the "acceptable" version and those who won't challenge us in our sin.

We can only keep up the tension and stress of "hiding" for so long. Deep within us is a cry for authenticity and consistency. So what keeps us so bound by our secrets? *Fear* . . . the fear of rejection, the fear of what the truth might require of you, and the fear of admitting how lost you truly feel.

To say out loud to another human being, "I had an abortion last year" or "My father molested me throughout my childhood" or "I can't stop looking at porn" would bring a reality to the pain that has been buried in your heart. If someone else knew, then you could no longer pretend.

After each question, circle who is responsible:

- **Who do you think is more invested in our hiding?**
  Satan or God?

- Who is it that whispers *They'll never accept you if they know!*
  Satan or God?

- Who invites us to step into truth instead of harboring our secrets?
  Satan or God?

God is not behind our hiding. He understands our shame and fear. He is a gentleman, not demanding that we tell our secrets, but inviting us to trust Him in the light. Jesus came to this earth to set us free—free from shame, free from the bondage of sin, and free from the power of our secrets.

The enemy knows that healing and freedom don't come in darkness but instead when we step into the light. While secrets have power, stepping into the truth can be even more life changing. I have had the privilege of being the person to whom secrets have been first spoken. Secrets of an addiction. Secrets of a shameful trauma. Secrets of a fantasy life no one knows about. When the words are whispered through tears and fear, a ray of light appears—light that gives hope.

The Bible may have been written thousands of years ago, but it contains stories of people just like us. King David is one of the heroes of the Bible. Even so, he was a great sinner and tried to hide his sin.

REFLECT AND RESPOND

- *Read Psalm 32:1-5. What was David's relationship with God like when he hid (or lied about) his sin?*

- *What did David do to "come out of hiding"?*

- *Read 1 John 1:8-9. What do these verses say is the difference between hiding sin and confessing it?*

If God Forgives, Why Don't I Feel Forgiven?

Yesterday, you read 1 John 1:8–9. These verses contain a promise. When we confess our sins, God will not only forgive us but also cleanse us from all unrighteousness. Do you believe that? I have met many women who nod their heads as if to say, "Yes, I believe that." But when I look at their lives, they are still burdened by their sin, especially their sexual sin. They still believe they have to do something to prove to God how sorry they are for messing up so badly.

> I am that woman who was going to wait until marriage but when I was thirty-five, I felt it was never going to happen and someone actually said that a woman could go through early menopause if they never had sex. I was scared. I wanted a family one day so the next few men I dated I did have sex with. I regret it now (I'm almost forty-one) and sometimes wonder, am I still not married because God is angry for what I did? —Candace

The truth is that we can confess our sins and ask God to forgive, yet still *feel* condemned and filled with shame because of our past sins and current struggles. I believe this is because Satan wants us to believe that we are beyond God's forgiveness. He tells us lies that make us feel as if other people can be free, but we never can be. And we have our own list of reasons why.

- *I should have known better. I grew up in a Christian home.*

- *I've been with more men than I can remember.*

- *I've had an abortion. I don't deserve forgiveness and freedom.*

- *What if I keep slipping right back into the same sin?*

Part of our confusion is rooted in not understanding the difference between guilt and shame. Because we often use these two words interchangeably, it can be difficult to tease out the difference. *Guilt is rooted in something we have done.* Feelings of guilt are healthy when they reflect our true state of guilt. Often our feelings of guilt don't correspond with the reality of our guilt. For example, while some women backstab, slander, and manipulate others without losing a wink of sleep over it, others can feel tremendous guilt for events that are completely outside of their control. Our feelings of guilt (or lack thereof) are not a reliable barometer for measuring the reality of our guilt.

While guilt is rooted in what we have done, shame is the condemnation of who we are. True guilt can lead to repentance and restoration, but shame looms like an oppressive cloud, separating us from knowing the love of Christ.

There is a reason so many Christian women hang on to the shame even though they know about God's total forgiveness. There is someone who does not want you to be free; his name is Satan. He does not want God to have the glory shone through the miracle of forgiveness. He would much rather Christians walk in a cloud of shame instead experiencing the freedom God offers through forgiveness. When you begin to experience shame, there are three things you can do to combat it. 1) Recognize the voice, 2) Remember the cross and 3) Declare the truth. We will hit on the first of these today and pick up the other two tomorrow.

Step 1: Recognize the voice Not only is Satan called the father of lies, he is also called the "accuser." His job description is to make you feel guilty. Revelations 12:10 tells us that Satan accuses us before God day and night. He wants you to stay stuck in shame because this will keep you from worshiping and intimately knowing God.

A big part of knowing God's voice is learning to discern between God's conviction and Satan's accusations. When you feel guilty about something, how do you know who is speaking to you? God convicts us of sin for the sake of leading us to freedom. Our enemy taunts us for the purpose of keeping us in bondage. Below is a chart to help you understand the characteristics of God's voice compared to Satan's.

GODLY CONVICTION	SATAN'S ACCUSATIONS
God convicts me of a specific wrong thought, attitude, or behavior.	Satan accuses me of being a bad person.
God calls me to confess my sins to Him and those I've offended.	Satan wants me to stay paralyzed in hiding.
God provides forgiveness and a new start.	Satan tells me I can never be free or pure.

God longs for you to know and receive His forgiveness for your past. Satan wants you to dwell on how bad you are. His "fiery arrows" (Eph. 6:16) make you doubt that God could or would completely forgive you. Satan will discourage you with thoughts like these: *What you did was so bad that, with a past like yours, you can never be a true Christian.* When you discern the condemning voice of your enemy, remember that God would never cover you with shame. His voice always offers freedom. "Where the Spirit of the Lord is, there is freedom" (2 Cor. 3:17).

REFLECT AND RESPOND

- *Think back on a time when you felt guilty. Write a short description of the situation.*

- *Knowing the characteristics of God's voice versus Satan's voice, who was speaking to you? How do you know?*

- *Next time you feel guilty, what questions can you ask yourself to determine whose voice it is?*

Embracing God's Forgiveness

Have you ever felt like Satan's words of accusations feel truer than God's words of forgiveness? Honestly, it's often easier for me to believe that I'm beyond God's love than to believe promises like this one is Psalm 103: "For as high as the heavens are above the earth, so great is his love for those who fear him; as far as the east is from the west, so far has he removed our transgressions from us" (Ps. 103:11–12).

Satan's accusations feel powerful because in one sense, they ring true. In our sinful state, we are not worthy of fellowship with God. I don't deserve God's forgiveness. As the Bible says, we have sinned and fall short of God's glory (Rom. 3:23). God's gift of forgiveness is a total supernatural reality that flies in the face of my human sense of justice. I should die for my sins, yet Jesus took my sin upon Himself. Paul wrote, "For the wages of [my] sin is death, but the gift of God [to me!] is eternal life in Jesus Christ our Lord" (Rom. 6:23).

Step 2: Remember the cross If it were not for Jesus' sacrifice on the cross, we would be forever burdened with the condemnation of sin. Satan desperately wants you to forget the supernatural power of the cross. He's happy for you to wear one around your neck or hang one in your house, as long as you don't remember that Jesus' death on the cross forever cancelled sin! "Therefore, since we have been justified through faith, we have peace with God through our Lord Jesus Christ" (Rom. 5:1).

When Satan accuses you of your past, remind him that your sins have been forgiven by God. You are free! You are forgiven!

While the world might encourage you to "stop being so hard on yourself," a Christian's understanding of being free from sin is much different. Our freedom is a gift; a debt has been paid on our behalf. In repentance and confession, we receive the amazing gift that Jesus died to give us. We are called to live as new creatures, no longer saddled with the sin of the past.

Step 3: Declare the truth In God's sight your sin no longer exists. He does not keep a record of your wrongs. Receiving forgiveness means acknowledging the reality that your sins have been paid for. God keeps no record of your wrongs, and He longs *for you* to tear up the mental or actual list you have of your sins. This is such an important truth, go back and underline it!

When you feel the sting of accusation and shame, what do you do? You pull out the enemy's fiery dart and throw it back at him. You refuse to believe his lies and you declare God's truth out loud, "There is no condemnation for me because I'm in Christ Jesus" (Rom. 8:1, paraphrase).

In the powerful passage about spiritual warfare, Ephesians 6, we are told to put on the armor of God and then to stand. In fact, we are encouraged to "stand" three times in those few verses (Eph. 6:11, 13, 14). Holding the shield of faith in our left hand and the sword of the Spirit, which is the Word of God, in our right hand, we stand. And just as Jesus did when Satan tempted Him (Matt. 4), we declare Scripture in response to Satan's taunts: "Satan, you don't want me to forgive myself or other people because you don't want me to be free. You want me to be in bondage. You are not going to outsmart me. I am familiar with your evil schemes."

When guilt whispers condemnation, what do you do? You worship your King, who forgave you and brought you out of darkness into His glorious light. And you sing His praises loudly! When you are refusing and resisting the fiery darts of the enemy, worship is a wall of protection around your soul. So worship, declaring the truth of God's great love for you!

REFLECT AND RESPOND

- *Is there a past sin that the "accuser" likes to throw in your face? What is it?*

- *Next time Satan brings this accusation up, what could you do to stand up against it?*

- *Write out a declaration statement you can use to resist the "accuser" and remember the cross.*

- *Is there a sin area in your life where God is calling you to confess, repent, and draw near to Him again?*

- *Take time in the next couple of days to be alone with God. During your time together, ask Him to reveal any unconfessed sin. As He brings sin to mind, write each down on paper and specifically confess them to God.*

- *Now write the words of 1 John 1:9 across your list of sins. As a symbol of His total forgiveness, tear the list up and throw it away.*

- *As you wrap up your time with God, open your Bible and read Romans 8:38-39 as well as Psalm 103:12. Spend a few minutes meditating on the truth from both passages.*

A New Identity

As we learned last week, our sexual temptations and past sins don't define us. Second Corinthians 5:17 says, "Therefore, if anyone is in Christ, the new creation has come: The old has gone, the new is here!"

The power of God's forgiveness in your life isn't just about heaven and hell. It also changes your entire identity here on earth. Another barrier between us and the Lord is that we hold on to our old identity and don't allow Him to change us completely.

God is offering you more than a fresh start or a clean slate; He is inviting you into a whole new identity. Let's be clear about who God wants you to become. A new identity does *not* mean wearing a super-spiritual mask, wearing a cross around your neck, or pretending to have an intimate relationship with God. Your new identity in Christ is about inviting Him to redeem your brokenness. It means being open with the Lord and allowing Him to turn your sinful heart into a loving heart.

A few years ago, I was reading a story from the gospel of Luke and God spoke some new truth into my heart. The story may be familiar to you. It's found in Luke 7:36–50. Take a few minutes to read this story for yourself.

As you probably gathered from reading, there is a woman who crashes a party at the home of a religious leader. Although we don't know her name, we learn quite a bit about this woman from this short passage. What I most want you to notice is how this woman's identity changed through her personal experience with Jesus.

REFLECT AND RESPOND

- *What did you learn about the woman from Luke 7:36-50?*

- *How is she like you? Unlike you?*

- *Why do you think she was so desperate to be near Jesus?*

- *Reread verse 39. What was this woman's reputation? How do you imagine she earned that reputation?*

- *Now reread verse 47. What new reputation did Jesus give her?*

- *At the end of the party, who do you think knew Jesus more intimately, the woman or the religious man who hosted the party?*

- *What do you think caused one of them to be near to God and the other person to remain distant?*

God has invited you to do this study, *Sex and the Single Girl*, not because He wants you to "clean up" your sex life. You can obey all of the Christian "rules" about sex, and still be very distant from God, locked in fear, and hindered by brokenness. God wants a relationship with you. He offers you complete freedom in forgiveness and the power to live with a new identity!

Here's what I've learned over the past several years, ministering to women on the topic of sexuality. Your sexuality is either drawing you closer to God or it is a barrier to true intimacy and fellowship with Him. For most women, the latter is true. Their shame, their hidden wounds, their vows to never trust again, and their secret sins keep God at arm's length. They may be getting along just fine on the surface, but they don't know Jesus Christ intimately.

I am still learning, growing, and being vulnerable with the Lord but I have great hope in knowing that He loves me more than I can imagine and wants to know me personally. As I become closer to the Lord and slowly begin to understand Him more it wells up in my heart that everyone needs to know this. Through the years the Lord has continued to give me a passion for women and sexual brokenness. I think this happened because I fully surrendered my story and sexual brokenness to the Lord. Although at first I was filled with shame and guilt, I realized that the Lord wants only the best for me. He wasn't harsh and judgmental but extended the most gracious and loving invitation to heal. Healing has been a journey and not a one-and-done thing for me, but on this journey I am learning so much about the Lord and His love for me. Things are not perfect in my life. I still struggle and have to remind myself daily that I am loved beyond measure by the Father. He chose to redeem me and make me free. I am reminded to put my trust in Him and that He has great plans for me. He knows my dreams and desires, and I know He will continue to meet my needs. No matter if I have good days or bad days, I remember this. Each day the Lord pours His unfailing love upon me, and through each night I sing His songs, praying to God who gives me life. —Vanessa

I've had the profound privilege of watching Jesus set women free from porn, restore a marriage after betrayal, bring healing to sexual wounds from childhood, and remove the cloud of shame from women who thought they could never be free from their sin. Each of these women know Jesus like they never could have before. They may have been Christians for decades, but there had always been a wall between them and God. By stepping into their wound, Jesus became more than a distant God. He became Redeemer, Comforter, Counselor, and Friend.

Why do I care about whether you go to counseling for your wounds or cry out for freedom from your past? Oh, friend. It's only because I want you to know Jesus. I want you to know that His friendship isn't reserved for the super spiritual. It is offered to anyone who wants to walk in the truth and to embrace Him. Paul wrote: "For though we live in the world, we do not wage war as the world does. The weapons we fight with are not the weapons of the world. On the contrary, they have divine power to demolish strongholds. We demolish arguments and every pretension that sets itself up against the knowledge of God, and we take captive every thought to make it obedient to Christ" (2 Cor. 10:3–5).

We wrote this study to tear down strongholds—those things that prevent women from intimately knowing God. As Paul wrote, this is a spiritual work that must be won with spiritual weapons. I have strongholds in my life, just as you have in yours. Oh, God, please tear them down so that we might know true intimacy with You!

REFLECT AND RESPOND

- *In what ways are you holding on to your old identity and not allowing God to change you completely?*

- *How will you respond to God's invitation to forgiveness, freedom, and a new you? What is one way you can bring your shame or hidden wounds before the Lord this week?*

- *Brainstorm a few action steps you can take to allow Jesus to tear down the strongholds in your life so you might know true intimacy with Him.*

PULLING IT ALL TOGETHER

Below are key truths you have read about this week that also answer the questions posed at the start of the week. Now is the time to ask yourself, "How much have I embraced this truth in my life?" After each statement, circle the number (1–5) that represents the power of this truth in your life.

• The main message of the entire Bible is God's plan to break down the barriers (i.e., sin) that stand between His holy love and the people He created to be His own.

1   2   3   4   5

• God does not endorse my hiding but the enemy does because he knows healing and freedom come when I step into the light.

1   2   3   4   5

• Sexual sin "sticks" to me in a different way than other sins because they are tied to every aspect of who I am. This doesn't mean that sexual sins are unforgivable though!

1   2   3   4   5

• I can recognize the difference between God's voice convicting me and Satan's voice condemning me.

1   2   3   4   5

• Receiving forgiveness means acknowledging the reality that my sins have been paid for. God keeps no record of my wrongs and longs for me to do the same.

1   2   3   4   5

- My three step plan to live in freedom is to (1) recognize the voice, (2) re-member the cross, and (3) declare the truth.

  1   2   3   4   5

- My new identity in Christ is about inviting Him to redeem my brokenness and allowing Him to change me completely.

  1   2   3   4   5

- Forgiving myself may bring about the breakthrough I have been looking for.

  1   2   3   4   5

Which truth did you rate the lowest? Write that truth on a 3x5 card (or on your phone) and look at it this week. Ask God to plant this truth in your heart.

Now What?

SELF-REFLECTION/DISCUSSION QUESTIONS

Looking Backward:

- How would you describe your view of sexuality when you first started this study?
- What did you find challenging/frustrating as you worked your way through this study? Did you resolve this issue? If so, how? If not, what steps will you take to resolve it?
- Did you have an "ah-ha" moment that powerfully impacted you? If so, when was that moment?

Looking Inward:

- What are a few ways you've developed or grown as a result of what you've learned?
- Of all the topics addressed in this study (boundaries, temptation, character, etc.), which do you feel you are strong in? Which do you feel you are weak in?
- In the area(s) you are weak in, what steps will you take to develop and strengthen them?

Looking Upward:

- What have you learned about God throughout these six weeks?
- What are a few ways God has spoken to your heart?

Looking Forward:

- What is your next step in living out what you've learned?
- What are a few practical tools you gained from this study that you can take with you into daily life?
- Are there Scripture verses that really stuck out to you that you'd like to commit to memory? If so, make a list of them and consider transferring them to a note card or your phone for continued meditation.
- What are a few principles on sexuality you can share with a friend or peer when the time is right?

- Can you think of a few friends or peers that you believe would really benefit from this study? Brainstorm names and pray about reaching out to them.
- What suggestion(s) would you give to someone starting this study that would help her get the most from it?

Notes

Week 1: Why Sexuality Matters

1. The Barna Group, "A New Generation of Adults Bends Moral and Sexual Rules to Their Liking," Barna, October 31, 2006, https://www.barna.com/research/a-new-generation-of-adults-bends-moral-and-sexual-rules-to-their-liking/.

Week 2: Embracing a Grand Design

1. "NTSB Releases Final Report on Investigation of Crash of Aircraft Piloted by John F. Kennedy Jr." National Transportation Safety Board, July 6, 2000, https://www.ntsb.gov/news/press-releases/Pages/NTSB_NTSB_releases_final_report_on_investigation_of_crash_of_aircraft_piloted_by_John_F._Kennedy_Jr.aspx.

2. Kenny Luck, "The Deadly Deception of Sexual Atheism in the Church," *Charisma Magazine*, October 7, 2014, http://www.charismamag.com/life/relationships/20385-the-deadly-deception-of-sexual-atheism-in-the-church.

3. See https://www.yourbrainonporn.com/.

Week 3: Sexuality and Your Character

1. Oswald Chambers, *The Philosophy of Sin: How to Deal with Moral Problems* (London: Marshall, Morgan & Scott, 1960).

Acknowledgments

The idea for this study came many years before the publication. Because I have not been single for many years, I needed help translating foundational truths about sexuality into the reality of single women. Chelsey Nugteren and Abby Ludvigson both contributed significantly to that effort.

Many others have spoken into this work, sharing their stories and insights. Thank you to Hannah Nitz, Hosanna Ramsdell, Jessa Crisp, Esther Allen, and Linda Dillow. I'm also grateful for the women who went through the pilot studies, helping us to make this resource more impactful. Judy Dunagan, Linda Joy Neufeld, Erik Peterson, and the rest of the Moody team, thank you for partnering with us to get tools into women's hands and truth into women's hearts.

About the Author

DR. JULI SLATTERY is a widely known clinical psychologist, author, speaker, and broadcast media professional. Juli's commitment to biblical principles, relatable style, and quick wit has made her a highly sought-after speaker. Juli is the cofounder with Linda Dillow of Authentic Intimacy, an international nonprofit designed to minister to women on topics concerning intimacy and sexuality. She has authored eight books, including *25 Questions You're Afraid to Ask about Love, Sex, and Intimacy*; *Sex and the Single Girl*; *Pulling Back the Shades* (coauthored with Dannah Gresh); *Surprised by the Healer* and *Passion Pursuit* (both coauthored with Linda Dillow); and *Finding the Hero in Your Husband*.

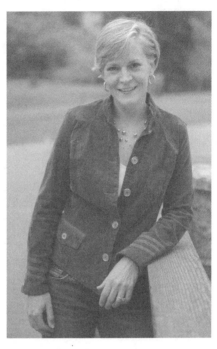

Dr. Slattery sits on the board of trustees for Moody Bible Institute. She hosts a weekly podcast called Java with Juli, and blogs regularly at authenticintimacy.com. Juli and her husband, Mike, have been married for over twenty years, have three boys, and live in Colorado Springs.

ABBY LUDVIGSON has been speaking and writing on the topic of sexuality for over a decade. You can follow her at sexbydesign.com. She and her husband, Greg, live in the outskirts of the Twin Cities area, where they enjoy the outdoors and all that country life has to offer.

CHELSEY NUGTEREN is a stay-at-home mom and freelance writer and marketer. She is passionate about God's design for marriage and family, and enjoys writing about her own journey as a wife and mom pursuing a life transformed by Jesus.

You wonder. Juli answers.

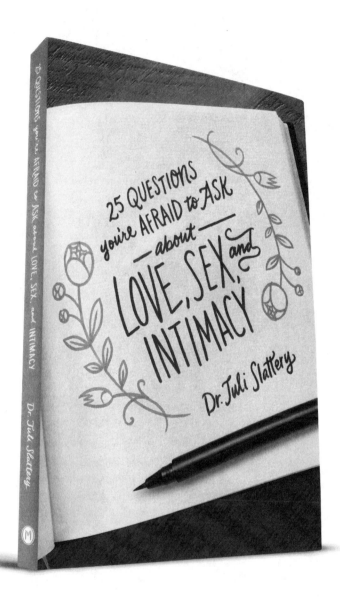

In this book, clinical psychologist Dr. Juli Slattery answers the most common and critical questions women ask her about sexuality, like *Can I be single and sexual? How do I know if he's the one? What do my temptations say about me?* Candid answers abound, freeing you to embrace God's design for love and sexuality.

978-0-8024-1342-0 │ also available as an eBook

You don't have to choose between being sexual or spiritual

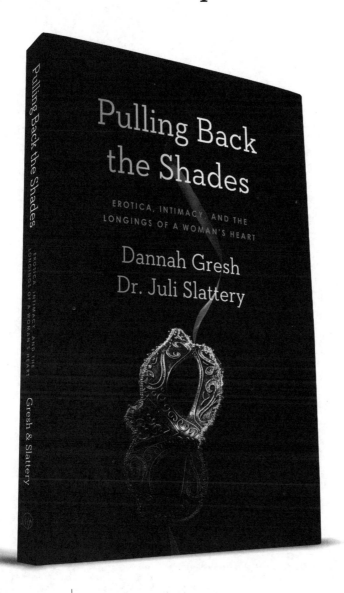

You don't have to stay broken.

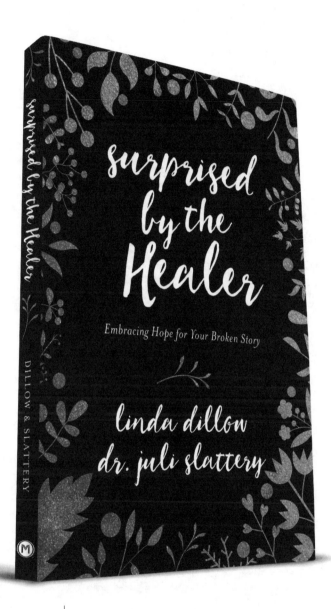

Java with Juli	

Searching for more?

Visit **javawithjuli.com** and subscribe to Dr. Juli Slattery's weekly podcast, *Java with Juli*, where she chats about sexuality, relationships, and intimacy with God.

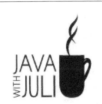